# The Validity of the Case Study

# American University Studies

Series XI
Anthropology and Sociology

Vol. 23

PETER LANG
New York • Bern • Frankfurt am Main • Paris

Daniel Leigh Haytin

# The Validity of the Case Study

## Deviance and Self-Destruction

PETER LANG
New York • Bern • Frankfurt am Main • Paris

**Library of Congress Cataloging-in-Publication Data**

Name: Haytin, Daniel Leigh, author.
Title: The validity of the case study:
deviance and self-destruction / Daniel Leigh Haytin.
Description: New York: Peter Lang, 1988.
Series: American university studies, series XI:
anthropology and sociology; v. 23 | ISSN 0740-0497
Includes bibliographical references and index.
Identifiers: LCCN 88012718 | ISBN 978-0-8204-0738-8 (hardcover: alk. paper)
Subjects: LCSH: Deviant behavior—Case studies.
Self-destructive behavior—Case studies. | Case method.
Classification: LCC HM291 .H39 1988 | DDC 302.5'42—dc19
LC record available at https://lccn.loc.gov/88012718

Bibliographic information published by **Die Deutsche Nationalbibliothek**.
**Die Deutsche Nationalbibliothek** lists this publication in the "Deutsche
Nationalbibliografie"; detailed bibliographic data are available
on the Internet at http://dnb.d-nb.de/.

The paper in this book meets the guidelines for permanence and durability
of the Committee on Production Guidelines for Book Longevity
of the Council of Library Resources.


29 Broadway, 18th floor, New York, NY 10006
www.peterlang.com



Printed in Germany

Dedicated to my parents,
Lois and Harold Haytin,
and to my sons,
Noah and Ari Haytin

## Contents

## Preface and Acknowledgements

This book represents many years of research on contrasting approaches—quantitative, qualitative and socio-psychoanalytic—to "deviant" and self-destructive behavior. It includes a case study of a young man who is a bisexual drug user, and who shall be given the pseudonym of "Dave." I first met Dave when we were classmates in junior high school in Los Angeles. We lost contact for many years until we met again in Berkeley, where I was a graduate student at the University of California. Upon hearing of my proposed research project, Dave eagerly agreed to be the "subject."

This book's treatment of the methodology of the case study is based upon both the interviews with Dave and my own research. The first two chapters are devoted to external considerations of method: the relationship between an audience's perceptions and the debate over the definition of what constitutes a "deviant" act, and geographical, historical, and political-economic influences on the audience's viewpoint. The final chapters will develop the specific case study of Dave.

I wish to express my sincere gratitude to Dr. James T. Carey, whose encouragement and academic guidance made this study possible. I am also indebted to professors William Smelser, Stanford Lyman, Edward Mooney, and Howie Clark for their intellectual inspiration and theoretical stimulation. Their insightful observations, perceptive suggestions and assistance in the conceptualization of the data in this book were exceedingly helpful.

—Daniel L. Haytin

# Chapter 1. Introduction

## I. A Brief History of the Case Study

The purpose of this book is to examine critically the validity of the case study as a methodological paradigm in the social sciences (specifically, psychology, sociology and criminology). The presentation has a tripartite design: consideration of methodological anomalies regarded by critics as inherent in case study method, a discussion of reactions by proponents of the method, and finally, a case study of multiple deviance.

Before examination and assessment of the case study's methodological validity, it will be helpful to discuss briefly the historical role of the case study in the social sciences. The use of case studies has traditionally been a part of the approach to all clinical research. Krafft-Ebbing (1881) and Lombroso (1891) employed case studies emphasizing autobiographical documents in their studies of social and psychological deviation. Kraepelin's recorded observations (1904) of mentally disturbed patients marked the beginning of psychiatric diagnostic classifications having their basis in case studies. This initiated the trend in psychology and psychiatry whereby case study method was used for descriptive, explanatory, and illustrative purposes.

As psychoanalytic theory emerged, the use of case study took on an exploratory role in which new hypotheses were discovered and generated. Each of Freud's case studies contained a discovery of either a special technique or a new theoretical insight. From the case studies of "Dora" (1925) and "Little Hans" (1926), Freud developed his techniques in the use of dreams. In the case of "The Rat Man" (1938), new obsessional neuroses—particularly the "Omnipotence of Thought"—were discovered. Freud distinguished different forms of repression from the case study of "The Psychotic Dr. Schreber" (1938), where the patient's autobiography was used, and developed techniques on transference and counter-transference from "The Wolf Man" (1944).

It is natural that this use of the case study method should originate in psychology and psychiatry, for the focus on the individual and the nature of the clinical setting, based on complex interpersonal relationships, discourages experimental methods. Etiological investigation and research into unknown areas involving intra-psychic subjective variables benefits from the use of case study method.

It was however Thomas and Znaniecki's voluminous work, "The Polish Peasant In Europe And America" (1927) which stimulated the interest of sociologists in this method. Thomas and Znaniecki based their investigation almost exclusively on personal documents—autobiographies, letters and newspaper articles—and upon exploration of the effects of industrialization, urbanization and ecological instability on the emigrating individual and his family. They believed that personal documents in the case study method "constitute the perfect type of sociological material."

Criminologists found life-history data such as biographies and interview records particularly valuable.

Healy and Brouner's (1945) case studies of youthful criminal offenders, Shaw's "The Jackroller" (1959) and Sutherland's "The Professional Thief" (1937) exemplify individualized criminological uses of the case study method. Collective uses of the case study method are typified by Thrasher's "The Gang" (1927) and by Whyte's "Street Corner Society" (1943). The case study became an invaluable methodology in the analysis of non-normative behavior and the etiological criminogenic study of "social deviations." It is at this point that the role and function of the case study underwent a critical methodological transformation.

In its prior usage in psychology and psychiatry, the case study was utilized as an exploratory, explanatory method often leading the way toward the development of new hypotheses and discoveries. Further usages were discouraged by the scientific objectivity required in experimental methodology. While most researchers in social science acknowledged this use of the case study for generation of hypotheses, few would recognize its use as a legitimate method for validation of hypotheses. Experimenters argued that it was not possible to generalize objectively from individual cases. Allport (1947, 1955, 1961) developed an opposing view which emphasized that the understanding of one single individual is a legitimate scientific goal and that the orientation of social scientists should be redirected toward this goal. Allport stressed the intrinsic subjectivity of human behavior and the irreducibility of human characteristics into quantifiable variables. This methodological controversy is perhaps one of the more salient areas to consider in the analysis of the case study's validity and will be discussed in later chapters.

## II. Definition of Terms

The term "case study" is an ambiguous one, encompassing a variety of connotations. Although it has its genesis in medicine, its modern day usage in clinical psychology is inherited from psychiatry. In its contemporary psychological usage, "case" is often designated as a human being who is suffering from a physical or emotional disorder. This usage is most commonly found at clinical staff conferences and implies a form of depersonalization harmful to the individual involved. It is worth noting that recently, many staff clinicians have replaced the words "case" and "patient" with "client" in order to avoid depersonalization.

For an accurate definition to be obtained, it is first necessary to understand the term "case study" as a composite term which derives its meaning from life or case histories, personal records, biograms, and human or personal documents. The above must be defined separately, for their usage in the literature is often confusing, and their theoretical conceptualizations are inter-related and inter-dependent.

Dollard (1935, 3), who emphasizes the cultural influences, defines a life history as a:

> Deliberate attempt to define the growth of a person in a cultural milieu and to make theoretical sense out of it.... From the standpoint of the life-history, the individual is viewed as an organic center of feeling moving through a culture and drawing magnetically to him the strands of the culture. In the end, the

> individual appears as a person, as a microcosm of the group features of his culture.

Drever (1963, 33) defines a "clinical life-history" as "a record of an individual's experience, illnesses, education, environment, behavior, and generally, all facts relevant to the particular problems involved in a medical or clinical case." Bolgar (1965, 28) explains the term "case-history" in its medical usage:

> Case-history originally meant the history of a patient's current illness or of several illnesses which added up to his medical history. Social scientists usually speak of the "life-history" of a person, and they refer to the data from which a life-history is culled as "personal documents." With the advent of the psychologist in the clinic, the case history became the medical as well as the social history of a person supplemented by personal documents and psychological test data.

Abel (1947, 11) limits his definition of a "personal record" to first person data only, "The term 'Personal Record' applies to any verbal or written information obtained from individuals about themselves. Personal records include reports of interviews, findings based on questionnaires, diaries, memoirs, case histories and sundry life-story documents." In an attempt to alleviate the ambiguity of terms, Abel differentiates his term "biogram" from autobiographies and life-histories by distinguishing between motivational factors. Whereas the motivational factor operating in the initiation of an autobiography or life-history is on an individualistic level, the motivational factor for a biogram is on a collective or group level. Both a life-history and an autobiography concern themselves with a particular individual who is either selected by a researcher, or initiated the data her or himself. Abel (1947, 114) contends that the term "autobiography" should be used restrictively, only when a life-story is initiated by its author, and intended as history or literature. For those life-stories written on request and intended to be used as data, the term "biogram" should be used. "Biograms are life-stories written on request by persons who are members of a selected social group, and in compliance with specific directions as to content and form for the purpose of obtaining mass data."

The terms "human document" and "personal document" are also used interchangeably, but their meanings are not quite as divergent as the terms "life-history," "case-history," "personal record" or "biogram."

Blumer (1939, 29) defines "human document" as "an account of individual experience which reveals the individual's actions as a human agent and as a participant in human life." Angell (1945, 177) broadens the parameters in his definition of a "personal document" to include third person interpretations, "For our purposes a personal document is defined as one reveals a participant's view of the experiences in which he has been involved. It is not absolutely essential that the individual whose conception of a situation is set forth should have written the document himself." Personal documents are defined by Bolgar (1965, 33) as first- or third-person accounts: "First-person documents include spontaneous communications, such as letters, diaries, and autobiographies; responses to interviews; free-association; communication of dreams and other matters made during the course of psychotherapy. Third-person accounts are biographies, including clinical case histories and systematic here-now observations of behavior."

Allport (1961, 401) stresses the intentionality variable and defines a "Personal Document" as:

> Any self-revealing record that intentionally or unintentionally yields information regarding the structure, dynamics, and functioning of the author's mental life. It may record the participant's view of experiences in which he has been involved; it may devote itself deliberately to self-scrutiny and self-description; or it may be only incidentally and unwittingly self-revealing. Among these would be included: (1) Autobiographies, whether comprehensive or topical; (2) diaries, whether intimate or daily log-inventories; (3) letters; (4) open-ended questionnaires (but not standardized tests); (5) verbatim recordings, including interviews, confessions, and narratives; (6) certain literary compositions.... It is important to note that these are all first-person documents. In addition to these, we have varieties of third-person records: case studies, life-histories, and biographies.

Angell and Freedman (1953, 302) bifurcate "personal documents" in expressive and non-expressive categories and describe the various types in each category, "Expressive documents (as opposed to non-expressive documents like court records, official histories and commissions' proceedings) are divided into A) personal letters, B) life-histories: either diaries, autobiographies, or what Abel (1947) calls biograms, and C) accounts of small group process."

Since all of the above terms (life or case-history, personal record, biogram, and human or personal document) deal exclusively with a single individual and are inextricably inter-related, they shall be incorporated under one topical category designated as the "case study" and will be analyzed together for their methodological validity. The term "case study" shall be operationally defined for this book as any form of first- or third-person expressive document that intentionally or unintentionally yields information regarding the structure, dynamics, and functioning of the actor's life (psychic and/or social), and attempts to describe in detail the actor's actions on a praxeological level. Also included is an extensive, comprehensive and unbiased account of the actor's life-history and a description of his/her Weltanschauung (i.e., values, beliefs, customs, reference groups, role identifications, and self conceptions). The case-study's data may be composed of information obtained from such expressive sources as artistic and projective productions (e.g., Rorschach, T.A.T., Draw-a-Person tests or paintings, and poems), letters, diaries (e.g., intimate journals, memoirs, and log-inventories), open-ended questionnaires, verbatim recordings (i.e., written or tape-recordings of interviews of dreams, confessions, and fantasies), autobiographies, and any other communicational medium or informational form which is self-revealing and self-disclosing.

By the term "praxeological," it is meant that the case study attempts to portray phenomenologically the actor's social and psychological world from the actor's reference point and strives to perceive and describe the existential meanings that the actor's actions hold for her or him. Thus, praxeology becomes an exercise in role-reversal and documenting reality as the actor perceives and interprets it—viewing the world through her/his eyes.

The phrase "extensive, comprehensive, and unbiased account of the actor's life-history" represents the case study's chronological documentation of all relevant social and psychological facts. This life-history information is of great importance for analyzing the impact of temporal and spatial variables in personality fluctuations. (The temporal and spatial dimensions shall be examined later.) The Goffmanic (1959, 123) meaning of "career" best conveys what is meant by:

> Extensive, comprehensive and unbiased life-history data ... any social strand of a person's course through life. The perspective of natural history is taken: unique outcomes are neglected in favor of such change over time as are basic and common to members of a social category, although occurring independently of them. Such a career is not a thing that can be brilliant or disappointing; it can be no more a success than a failure.

The terms "self-revealing and self-disclosing" mean that the case study researcher includes an analysis of the actor's communicative actions. Every communicative act, whether gestural, verbal or written, conveys a projection of the actor's socio-psychological self. "No matter what else human beings are communicating about, they are always communicating about themselves, about one another, and the immediate context of the communication" (Pittengner et al. 1960, 229). Therefore, "communicational medium or informational form which is self-revealing and self-disclosing" should be interpreted by the reader as the case study's dramatization of the actor's phenomenological self by analyzing her/his communicative acts. Jourard (1964, 24) illustrates this, "I don't mean anything mysterious by 'Self.' All I mean is the person's subjective side—what he thinks, feels, believes, wants, worries about—we get to know the other person's self when he discloses it to us." Jourard believes self-disclosure is the portrayal of one's soul through the communication of one's self to another. The case study incorporates and displays the actor's self.

# Chapter 2. Alleged Methodological Anomalies and Invalidities

The case study method has received most criticism over its reliance on subjective accounts which are derived from single cases. The case study is built upon subjectivity, compiling its information from such sources as human and personal documents, biograms, and case-histories. Thus, the case study method is viewed by many as unscientific because of its lack of methodological objectivity. Rosenzweig (1948, 575) writes:

> The case history method has frequently been criticized as unreliable and consequently, unscientific as a method of approach in the study of human behavior. These criticisms have been based on two important observations. First, the report depends on the memory or recall of past events of either the client or informant, and recall is known to be inaccurate, especially when one is asked to recall events of several years previous. Second, any report is likely to be given with either a "Halo Effect" or with a bias, and consequently it may be either consciously or unconsciously distorted.

Angell and Freedman (1953, 306) list the case-study's methodological anomalies and deficiencies as, "1) The optimum scope of a study by this means is limited. 2) The unrepresentativeness of the document. 3) The unreliability of the record. 4) The unreliability of the analyst's interpretations of the record. 5) The validity of the findings is unassessable."

The methodological anomalies attributed to the paradigmatic use of case study in the social sciences can best be evaluated if divided into two major categories: (A) lack of objectivity as a scientific product; and, (B) problems in understanding the full significance in generalizations of particular cases encountered by those without first-hand knowledge of them.

The first category consists of a multitude of interrelated sub-categories, the first anomaly of which is concerned with the lack of data-control and the unreliability of information. This anomaly suggests that the primary source of data upon which a case study is developed is unreliable, and therefore the study is invalidated. Here, critics question the credibility, motivation and reliability of the author of personal documents and biograms.

Another criticism of data sources lies in a lack of investigative control over the form, structure and direction of the data. The research investigator receives, at second or third hand, information which has been composed independently of his influence. This proposed anomaly regarding information control by social science researchers is discussed by Angell and Freedman (1953, 300):

> Documents, census materials, and indices characteristically bring the data to the social scientist in a form over which he has little control. In contrast, when the social scientist uses the method of observation, either participant or non-participant, he can focus on those

> aspects of the behavior of the subject that have theoretical interest for him; if he uses tests and questionnaires, he chooses to frame the instrument to suit his scientific needs; during the interview, the Subject may be guided by the interviewer, and if crucial points are unclear, the interviewer can probe until the matter is elucidated. Although there are exceptions, documents, records and indices come ready-made; some other person, either a participant in a social situation or process, the originator of a system of recording, or the creator of an index, determines the form of the data.

Therefore the data of the case study is characteristically based on information (communication or observation of events) which was not intended for the social scientist (unless specifically motivated by the researcher).

Criticism concerning lack of control over the original information displays its weakness when one considers that the lack of the researcher's control and influence upon the data results in a "purification" of the data. Raw data is "pure" when it has been produced solely on the basis of individual motivation. Hence, its validity is increased rather than decreased when the originator of the information is ignorant of the social scientist's theoretical orientation and biases. If an author writes a document or biogram without any influence from the researcher, then his information yields an unbiased product. In light of the author's ignorance of the social scientist's research intentions and needs (and thus producing unbiased data) the informational control anomaly is specious in its consequences. The "purity" of the data is determined directly by the author's intention or motive for creating the information.

The motivational factor must be considered prior to an assessment of an author's reliability and credibility. There are myriad motivations which will cause the author to produce a document or biogram. Krueger and Reckless (1935, 578) suggest that all personal documents can be classified as either "confessional," or "detached." Shaw and Burgess (1930, 205) broaden the distinctions into a four-fold classification: "Chroniclers," "Self-defenders," "Confessants," and "Self-analysts." Gottschalk (1945), Garrety (1957) and Allport (1961) have enumerated the possible motivations as exhibitionism, scientific interest, desire for immortality, justification and excuse, redemption and social re-incorporation, monetary gain, catharsis and exorcism, atonement, deception and fraudulent misrepresentation. Interdependently related to the motivational factor is the factor of the audience toward which the communication was directed. There is a qualitative difference in validity assessment between first- and third-person accounts and the form of the communication. A diary is often aimed at a fantasized audience whereas a letter is directed at an audience whose identity is known to the author. Certainly the audience toward which the document is directed will alter the form and nature of the content.

Veracity, credibility and reliability must be adduced with other factors in mind, such as motivation, purpose, intent and external influence—a researcher's instructions. Many documents which were motivated by the request of a researcher will contain invalid information. Authors and informants may deliberately misrepresent and falsify their information either to "put on" the researcher, appear impressive, or to rationalize, justify, emphasize, neutralize or excuse their actions. They may skew their information towards their concept of the researcher's orientation and hypothetical goals (assumptions). For example, if the interviewee perceives the interviewer as mainly interested in drug usage, s/he may disproportionately discuss his drug usage.

Many personal documents are motivated deliberately by a desire to deceive. Allport (1947, 130) states, "Specious statements within personal documents range in type from unconscious rationalizations to deliberate hoaxes." Also, an honest error may be present which produces misinformation. An author or informant may make an unconsciously motivated error of memory or perception in attempting to recall past experiences and events. Erroneous testimonies, either accidental and unintentional or, deliberate deceptions perpetrated by authors and informants, therefore constitute invalid, fallacious data.

This anomaly is based on the assumptions that (1) misrepresentation, deception and falsification, either by design or by accident is undetectable by the researcher, and that (2) an informant's accidental misrepresentation or deliberate attempt to deceive totally invalidates his/her information.

The weaknesses in the former assumption are pointed out in a later section, (Nomothetic vs. Idiographic Conceptualization) under the criteria for the validation of a document's data. The latter assertion denies the entire philosophy and rationale which underlies case study method: the uniqueness of subjectivity and the individualistic, idiosyncratic nature of human beings. Case study bases its virtue and strength as a legitimate methodology in the social sciences on the diversification and relativity of human existence. Determining what is "objective truth," "absolute truth" or "universal truth" is phenomenologically impossible and is, in fact, the goal and major purpose of the case study—to arrive at the actor's definition of truth or reality as he sees it. As Shaw (op. cit., 55) has concluded:

> It is essential to deal with his (the actor's) personal attitudes, his definition of the situation although these may be exaggerations or even misrepresentations of the objective situation. Even if it were true that (the actor's) interpretations of the family situation were somewhat exaggerated, it cannot be doubted that he acted "as if" these interpretations were true.

Truth, in this case, is relative to the actor involved and is determined by his perception, his interpretation of his perceptions and his belief that something is true or untrue. Truth can thus be defined for the case study as "something the actor believes to be true." Consequently, truth becomes "objectified" by viewing it within the actor's frame of reference, unless he is consciously misrepresenting his account. If he is, then the misrepresentations, fabrications and exaggerations should be analyzed and interpreted as to the significance and meaning they have for the actor. In this way, the deliberate falsifications and distortions become validated and objectified by demonstrating the subjective meanings they hold for the actor. This is the very essence of the ethnomethodological and praxeological perspectives.

Gottschalk (1945, 35) in his discussion of the role truth plays in the establishment of historical fact, contends that it is the portion or *degree* of truth that is important in lieu of "totality of truth":

> That the particular datum within the document rather than the document as a whole is the subject of the historian's critical analysis and that credibility and verisimilitude rather than truth is its end. What is historical fact? In the process of analysis the chief question the historian asks is: Is this particular credible? It might be well to point out again that what is meant by credible is not that it actually happened as one can learn from a critical examination of the best sources available. The historian thus establishes credibility and verisimilitude rather than truth.

Following Gottschalk's line of reasoning, the goal of the methodological investigator should be to determine the credibility of the document's significant portions rather than analyzing it as a whole. A document can be entirely false, yet contain a significant amount of credible information.

Freud, for example, through realizing the relativity and subjectivity of truth, revised his original theory concerning the etiology of neurosis. He felt the genesis of neurosis lay in early childhood experiences involving a seduction by an older relative or parent-surrogate. Later, he discovered, through intensive self-analysis and reasoning (the reported frequency of sexual acts by adults against his analysands was incredible) that it was practically impossible for him to distinguish between objective realities and unconsciously precipitated fantasies. At this "discovery" Freud (1924) noted feeling "more triumph than defeat" and was lead to revise and reformulate (1896b) his original hypothesis:

> This section was written while I was under the ascendancy of an error which I have since then repeatedly acknowledged and corrected. I have not yet found out how to distinguish between patients' fantasies about their own childhood and real memories. I consequently ascribed to the etiological factor of seduction an importance and general validity it does not possess.

Freud's insight resulted in monumental consequences for psychological theory: out of this emerged his "discovery" of the Oedipus Complex as an etiological base for neurosis.

Clearly the information presented to Freud could not have been less reliable as to fact, yet it enabled him to gain new insights and to hypothesize new theoretical constructs. First-person personal documents (such as letters, autobiographies and diaries) may also be filled with misrepresentations and fantasies, yet their validity as documents is not decreased, but increased with proper processing of the data by researchers.

Another classic example of how sociological and psychological theories and clinical advances emerge from untrustworthy sources is found in Clifford Beers' (1938) biography, "A Mind That Found Itself." Beers wrote his autobiography shortly after recovering from what was diagnosed as a manic-depressive breakdown which needed months of institutional treatment. Even while writing, Beers still suffered from a mild form of the psychosis. This personal document failed practically all validating criteria: it utilized no independent sources of information, it failed to corroborate its facts with outside variables, it failed to assess the representativeness of the character of the experience, it failed to analyze its information as a comprehensive extensive basis, and its scope was limited to the experience of a single individual (ignoring demographic data and life history information). However, in spite of all the document's methodological limitations and deficiencies, its psychological and sociological contributions are monumental. This document is regarded as directly responsible for founding the mental hygiene movement in America and, through exposing the many evils of contemporary institutions, helped to initiate humanitarian reform of institutional policies. Few documents could be more "invalid" from the point of view of data control and authenticity, yet this document (which has gone through three translations) has been credited with innumerable contributions to psychiatry and to psychopathology, and is regarded as a classic in mental sciences.

Autobiographies supply the investigator with expressive, first-person accounts which can only be communicated through the author's perception and interpretation of what he sees. The concept of "metho-dological validity," vis-a-vis the writing of an autobiography, is often irrelevant and inapplicable. The autobiographer's experiential communications are valuable however, for they provide researchers with unique and individualistic data which originates in otherwise inaccessible times, places and psychic states. Hence, new and different areas of life experiences are opened up for systematic exploration.

Researchers have been stimulated by a multitude of such first-person personal documents. Prominent examples are: Anonymous (1921) and Buhler's (1934) intensely personal experience of adolescence; Frankl (1946), Wiesel (1967) and Bettelheim (1960) on concentration camps; Hachiya (1955) on surviving thermonuclear war; Beers' autobiography on mental illness (1939); Keller (1903) on mastery of physical handicaps; Byrd (1938) and Burney (1952) on social isolation; Sarton, Gollwitzer et al. (1956) on aging and imminent death.

While autobiographies are rich in information which would be otherwise unobtainable, letters constitute the most readily available form of first-person personal documents. Letters have contributed vast amounts of dyadic communications which in turn have supplied the necessary information for invaluable case studies. Yet letters are unquestionably subjective and unreliable communications. Despite their non-empirical character, letters are used continually by social science researchers in a multitude of forms. Perhaps their most celebrated use is found in Thomas and Znaniecki's monumental work, "The Polish Peasant In Europe and America" (1927) where 764 letters were utilized. Their work can be analyzed as a prototypical example of the inherent methodological anomalies and deficiencies in validity attributed to the use of letters.

Blumer (1939, 36) criticized Thomas and Znaniecki's personal documents for failing, upon individual examination, to meet any of the four criteria of his evaluation: their representativeness is not established; their adequacy for the motivational purpose for which they are employed is not analyzed; their reliability is not corroborated by independent sources; and the validity of interpretations derived from any single document is not demonstrated. Although the four criteria of scientific acceptability were not met, it is important to note that Blumer hastens to add, "To set aside the documents as having no scientific value would be to ignore the understanding, insight and appreciation which their careful reading yields." He concludes that taken collectively, their methodological validity is also increased by presenting a more comprehensive and consistent perspective; that by their vast numbers, the documents' representativeness, adequacy and reliability are greatly improved. (The methodological validity of single cases and single personal documents is examined in a later section.)

Thomas and Znaniecki's work contains another methodological anomaly in that their documents present only one side of the communication. Ideally, letters should represent the entire communication process between sender and recipient. Dyadic relationships are more adequately analyzed when the interactional data of both sender and receiver is chronologically presented. The fact that only one side of the communication is presented coupled with the intrinsic subjectivity of letters, significantly limits methodological validity. Where data is unidimensional due to its unavailability, the result is a fragmentary and incomplete representation. Even with this limiting deficiency, Thomas and Znaniecki's work can be validated and objectified by applying methodological models of quantification schemes, such as Parsons' "Pattern Variables" (1953), Boles' "Code" (1950), Le Play's "Explanatory Supplements" (1879), Baldwin (1940), and Sussman's "Systematic Content Analysis of Letters" (1956).

All of the letters, (except those which "contained nothing but a repetition of situations and attitudes") are published, and every interpretation and theoretical inference by Thomas and Znaniecki is footnoted directly to the letter. This enables the reader to assess exactly which particular phrases, paragraphs, and passages result in specific interpretations. By presenting all relevant data available and by correlating theoretical inferences and hypotheses with particular portions of the data, a reader can readily adduce anomalous methods. In analyzing Thomas and Znaniecki's use of letters, Riley (1963, 243) concludes:

> In contrasting the use of letters with the methods of observation and questioning let us emphasize again that the data used here were not produced originally for purposes of research. The letters are the interaction in a form even more genuine than the interaction artificially induced in the laboratory. Thus, these data are free from the potential errors that so often beset the observer or the questioner—the errors of control effect, and (when the letters are in their complete and original form) the errors of biased-viewpoint effect. The preconceptions of the investigator cannot affect what the group members actually write to one another, nor is there any opportunity for selective reporting by the researcher.

Other case studies which have employed letters have included the data from both the sender and recipient. Letters may not reveal all facets of a single personality but they do reveal the socio-psychological nexus which links the two personalities. Kahle's (1931) investigation analyzed the incoming and outgoing letters of two hundred institutionalized females. The letters provided information concerning the different kinds of relationships between the women and their families and also revealed the effects of absence as the degree of idealization of the relationships. Perry (1935) constructed the character and thought of William James on the basis of the latter's extensive correspondence.

Interpersonal dyadic relationships must be analyzed on an interactional-transactional level, including the actions and reaction of both parties. This diminishes the relative distortions of the data which occur due to audience expectations, over-reactions and misinterpretations. Jones (1935), while analyzing Freud's correspondence, found there was a great deal of difference in the content of the letters, even when scientific points were discussed, depending upon the person receiving the letter. Jones studied Freud's letters on a longitudinal level and discovered that while his earlier letters were written to alleviate tension, his later ones were concerned with helping his friends.

Correspondence over a long period of time offers invaluable data for the study of such variables as attitudinal and identity fluctuation, maturation and the aging process. Bolgar (1935, 34) studied more than two thousand letters which covered the adult life of three individuals and has traced the transitions and changes in goals, needs and values through their correspondence. Bolgar feels:

> The use of letters has made it possible to learn about thoughts, feelings and spontaneous concerns of the authors at the actual time of experience and to observe the changes connected with maturation and aging. No other type of personal document provides such immediate here-now, first-hand reporting continued over long periods of time.

William James' (1907, 147) pragmatic theory of truth most accurately describes the intrinsic weakness of this anomaly which suggests that the case study method is invalid due to distortions and errors of documental information. James professed that:

> An idea is "true" so long as to believe it is profitable to our lives. "Truth" in our ideas and beliefs means the same thing that it means in science. It means nothing but this, that ideas (which themselves are but parts of our experience) become true just insofar as they help us to get into satisfactory relation with other parts of our experience—that all our true ideas are useful and all those of ideas which are useful, are true. Theories thus become instruments, not answers to enigmas in which we can rest.

Pragmatic truth is that form of truth which is operating in the formulation of case studies. That is, information is "true" or valid when it is functional, useful and valuable. The data contained in personal documents, biograms, human and/or life-histories becomes valid when perceived in this pragmatic and utilitarian perspective. Methodological validity (or truth) is obtained when the author of the case study determines first, the motivational factor initiating the production of the information, and second, the underlying subjective meaning the communication contains for its originator.

In addition to the "data control anomaly," critics believe the case study method to be invalid and unscientific because of its methodological reliance upon single cases, its author's implicit and arbitrary conceptualizations, and its lack of standardized and codified measurements.

By definition, case study method deals exclusively with a single individual. The personal documents which provide the raw data for case studies also deal with single individuals. First and third-person documents find themselves in one common methodological quandary: they both deal with the *single case* and on this question they will stand or fall together (Allport 1947, xiii).

The central methodological issue is illuminated by Bolgar (1959, 135):

> In spite of its venerable history and undeniable contribution to psychological theory, the case study method is a controversial issue and is often referred to as *pre*-scientific rather than scientific, particularly by researchers whose major commitment is to hypothesis validation rather than hypothesis generation. While this may be an artificial dichotomy, and while many researchers cross lines or attempt to combine the two commitments, there are differences between the two attitudes. These differences appear with regard to the problems of data collection, rigorousness of design and interpretation of the data. It is probably appropriate to consider the clinical researcher who is primarily committed to the case study approach as a "naturalist" in perhaps somewhat artificial contrast to the experimentalists.

Bolgar's dichotomy may be artificially imposed upon researchers, but in examining the nomothetic and idiographic approaches, it appears a very useful dichotomy. The nomothetic approach (which includes "objectivists," "empiricists," "experimentalists," and "hard data quantifiers") dictates that theoretical generalizations should be applicable to *many* individuals, and derives the generalizations through systematic experimentation, usually involving the use of statistical validation. Nomothetists usually credit the case study with being an excellent didactic aid in learning theoretical constructs in the social sciences and also function to generate new discoveries. Beyond this acknowledgement however, the uses and contributions of the case study diminish as the nomothetists insist that it is scientifically impossible to generalize from single cases.

The idiographic approach (the adherents of which include "naturalists," "subjectivists," and "soft data investigators") stresses the legitimacy of investigating and researching the life of a single individual and is only secondarily concerned with the frequency or nature of a variable outside the realm of that individual's life. This view contends that it is scientifically valid and methodologically correct to study the behavior of one human being and to perceive him not only as a representative of a group, but also as an independent totality from whom generalizations can be formulated.

The underlying philosophy of the idiographic point of view, which derives its rationale from uniqueness and individuality, is described by James (1902, 10):

> The first thing the intellect does with an object is to class it along with something else. But any object that is infinitely important to us and awakens our devotion feels to us also as if

> it must be *sui generis* and unique. Probably a crab would be filled with a sense of personal outrage if it could hear us class it without ado or apology as a crustacean, and thus dispose of it. "I am no such thing" it would say, *"I am myself, myself alone."*

The idiographic approach to the study of human behavior contends that the true goal of the social sciences is *understanding* behavior, not merely quantifying, classifying or dissecting it. The conflict between the idiographic and nomothetic approaches boils down to, as Bryman (1984) points out, an epistemological question. Giddens (1976) and Bleicher (1982) agree that in contrast to the nomothetic approach, the idiographic approach does not try to break what Charles Taylor (1971) refers to as the "hermeneutic circle," the level of ambiguity, and the conflict of interpretation present in any idiographic analysis of data. Rather, the nomothetic approach seeks to break the circle in two ways: (1) it "aspires to attainment of an understanding of such clarity that it would carry with it the certainty of the undeniable"; and (2) to "reconstruct knowledge in such a way that there is no need to make final appeal to readings or judgements which cannot be checked further" (op. cit., 29). Both attempts are rooted in the assumption that quantification, rather than interpretation, concretizes the data in such a way as to meet the two requirements set out above. This assumption is false—false because quantification is artificial, a human artifact, and in the final analysis, only another form of interpretation, albeit one that uses the notation (numbers) of the natural sciences and thus appears certain and permanent. (Cf. Bogdan & Steven Taylor

1975; Barroch & Silvers 1982.) In short, the idiographic approach, even with all of its uncertainties, does not delude itself in a false quest for a certainty that cannot exist. An idiographic analysis results in detailed understanding rather than abstract and meaningless numbers.

Because of the uniqueness and individuality of personalities, understanding of human behavior is best achieved through case study method. Idiographists believe personalities are so unique, idiosyncratic and varied, that the most valid method of studying behavior is case study method whereby the entire personality is explored at a Gestaltist level.

Rosenzweig (1948, 575) discusses the significance of personality variability in the psychological use of case study method:

> The definition of personality has come to involve at least two indispensable ideas: integration and uniqueness. While other aspects of psychological research are directed to this or that segment of behavior, personality invariably refers to the functioning of the whole man, and those aspects of integration that distinguish any individual from his fellow. In studying personality, the psychologist is therefore interested in knowing how the individual, in the expression of his needs and his relationships with other individuals, functions as a recognizable unit that possesses certain distinctive traits, drives, attitudes and habits, and attains, or fails to attain, an

> adjustment to himself and his environment. Perhaps the most important single instrument in the clinical examination is the case history. It is the only method by which the psychologist can gain an understanding of the development of the behavior. Psychological insight into the nature of any problem can be gained only by a knowledge of the forces in their chronological relationships, which have acted upon the individual and to which he has reacted to make him what he is.

Sperle (1933, 11) stresses the necessity of analyzing the totality of the personality:

> Personality signifies not only all that is native and individual to man, but all that comes to him by way of education, experience, and human intercourse. Our physical heredity, our innate qualities transmitted and unalterable are individual; all that portion of our social heritage and our environment which we have been able by day-to-day living to add to individuality and make part of ourselves is personal; and the whole becomes our personality ... while a man's individuality does not change, his personality which includes both his native and acquired qualities, is forever changing.

Human behavior is contingent upon individual personality which in turn is contingent upon external phenomena—verbal and non-verbal communication, primary and secondary group identification and interpersonal relationships, sub-cultural and societal mores, and role expectations.

The statement, "only change is constant" is especially relevant in studying personality. Freudians often overstress the importance of early childhood and, at the same time, often underestimate the influence of adult experience. Social pragmatists, symbolic interactionists, phenomenologists, role theorists, stigma and labeling theorists (James, Marx, Dewey, Thomas, Mead, Schutz, Becker, Sarbin, Turner and Goffman) all emphasize the social derivation of the self; personality is a direct product of the actor's social world. An individual's personality (self-concept or ego-identity) is thus socially bestowed and so subject to external sociological forces. Changes in sociological milieu will effect changes within an individual's personality. These sociological changes may be real or imagined and still significantly alter a personality. The changes can be as superficial as sporting a new ensemble or as drastic as leaping from a building during the stock market crash.

Erikson's (1959) statement that, "Identity is never gained nor maintained once and for all" but is a dynamic, fluid and flexible phenomenon corresponds exactly to Becker's statement (1956, 523) that "Adult identity is a function of career movements within occupations and work organizations." Sarbin (1964) substantiates the continually fluctuating and alternating quality of the personality by demonstrating the interdependence of social roles with self-conceptions. Sarbin views social identity as simply all the statuses or positions an individual successfully occupies either through ascribed or achieved means. Every social role contains specified expectations, emotions, attitudes and actions which determine the character of the actor's personal identity. Through the process of social mobility, an actor constantly acquires new self-conceptions and personality traits. Berger (1963, 97) describes the personality changes accompanying changes in social roles:

> A man recently commissioned as an officer, especially if he came up through the ranks, will at first be at least slightly embarrassed by the salutes he now receives from the enlisted men. Probably he will respond to them in a friendly, almost apologetic manner. The new insignia on his uniform are at that point still something of a disguise. Indeed, the new officer may even tell himself and others that underneath he is still the same person, that he simply has new responsibilities (among which, *en passant* is the duty to accept the salutes of enlisted men). This attitude is not likely to last very long. In order to carry out his new role of officer, our man must maintain a certain bearing. This bearing has quite definite implication. Every military salute given by an inferior rank is an act of obeisance. Thus, with every salute given and accepted, (along, of course, with a hundred other ceremonial acts that enhance his new status) our man is fortified in his new bearing—and in its, as it were ontological presuppositions. He not only acts like an officer, he feels like one. Gone are the embarrassments, like the apologetic attitude, the I'm-just-another-guy grin.

Likewise a sage, beginning by acting wise, soon feels wise; the preacher comes to believe what he preaches and the comedian finds his material humorous. The experience of adolescence and pubescence indicates how far physiological changes—body image and physiognomy—can influence a personality.

Another example of the dynamic nature of personality and its dependence on social structures is the proselytization process. Through this process identities are transformed when an individual re-experiences himself on completion of a conversion ceremony. Large social structures and total institutions are responsible for re-creating and transforming personalities. Anything from joining the Black Muslims to joining a Kibbutz may have this effect. The transformation of an individual's identity is governed, as is its genesis and maintenance, by social processes which are potentially endless in their operation. Personality is never static *or* sustained, but is a metamorphosis passing through innumerable stages.

An individual's personality or identity, viewed in this perspective demands the comprehensive, extensive and in-depth analysis of the idiographic case study method for a valid understanding of human behavior. The inherent uniqueness and mutability of the human personality requires the idiographist's personalized and subjective approach. The idiographic approach is especially valuable as a methodological paradigm in connection with the phenomenon of functional equivalence and multi-causality. Allport (1961, 57) states, "What the nomothetist finds hard to contemplate is the very real possibility that no two lives are alike in their motivational processes." Functional equivalence deals with the multiplicity of motivational factors and demonstrates how a heterogeneous set of motives can manifest themselves in one homogeneous event. This phenomenon of functional equivalence, or multi-causality, has also been referred to as the polygenicity of simultaneous events. William James (1902, 399) in his discourse on the myriad existential experiences of life conjectured, "So many men, so many minds: I imagine that these experiences can be as infinitely varied as are the idiosyncrasies of individuals." A Roman aphorism runs, *si bis idem faciunt, non idem est* (if two people do the same thing, it is not the same thing). More simply, what is ostensibly an identical behavioral variable, in actuality could be the product of a galaxy of independent motivational variables. As Matza (1964) indicates, juvenile delinquency can be an end product of numerous motives—there are social, economic, psychological and political delinquents. Functional equivalence necessitates the study of behavior to include an individualistic, situational and circumstantial frame of reference.

Devereux (1961, 227) demonstrates how differing psychological motives yielded functionally equivalent sociological results during the Hungarian Revolution:

> Where one man revolts because he had been exploited, another will because, twelve years earlier, the Russians had raped his wife, another because he hates all authority, and still another may revolt because he wishes to

> impress his girlfriend with his patriotism and valor. All these men may fight with equal ardor, kill an equal number of secret police and Russians and therefore achieve militarily and socially identical results.

Psychologists are aware that a valid diagnosis could not be made on a single interview. It is known that an individual's present mood will greatly influence and often determine his statements. A subject experiencing an exceedingly depressed, pessimistic mood will perceive, interpret and communicate his data very differently than he would in a second interview when he is experiencing a cheerful mood. The influence of the subjective present on perception is perhaps universal amongst people. If one views human existence as comprised of past, present and future, then it is essentially only the present in which one exists. The existential present therefore has assumed disproportionate importance. As Berger (1963, 56) asserts:

> It is too easy to think that our own age is the epitome of what man has achieved so far, so that any past period can be judged on a scale of progress in terms of its closeness to or distance from the point at which we now stand. Perhaps the most decisive event of man's history on this planet took place on a quiet afternoon in the year 2405 B.C. when an Egyptian priest woke up from his siesta and suddenly knew the final answer to the riddle of human existence—and promptly expired without telling anyone. Perhaps everything that has

happened since is nothing but an inconsequential postlude.

It is impossible to calculate or to determine accurately the degree of situational and circumstantial influence on information received. Temporal and spatial dimensions are integral determinants of an individual's self concept and identity, which in turn, will determine the content of self-information collected. Berger (1963, 60) dramatically portrays the temporal-spatial influences on perception and interpretation:

> Social mobility has as monumental consequences in terms of the reinterpretation of one's life as does geographic mobility. Take the way in which man's self image is changed as he moves up the social ladder. Perhaps the saddest aspect of this change is the way in which he now interprets his relationships to the people and events that used to be closest to him. For example, everything connected with the Little Italy of one's childhood undergoes a malevolent mutation when viewed from the vantage point of the suburban home that one has finally clawed one's way to. The girl of one's teenage daydreams is transmuted into an ignorant though pretty peasant. Boyhood friendships become irritating reminders of an embarrassing former self, long left behind, together with old ideas of honor, magic and street corner patriotism. Even Mama, who used to be the orb around which the universe revolved, has become a silly old Italian

> woman one must pacify, occasionally, with a fraudulent display of an old self that no longer exists.

The idiographic approach of case study method analyzes human behavior on an in-depth, historical level which the nomothetic approach ignores. Information which is obtained without related and independent variables accounting for temporal and spatial influencing factors is inconclusive and incomplete. Goffman (1956, 123) recognizes this methodological anomaly in his analysis of the careers of mental patients:

> Here is a very ticklish point for the sociology of careers. An important aspect of every career is the view the person constructs when he looks backward over his progress; in a sense, the whole of the pre-patient career is derived from this reconstruction.

The state Governor, at age forty-five, either being interviewed or writing a personal document, will certainly assess and communicate his political life differently than he would twenty-five years earlier when he led a college strike as a campus radical.

Nomothetists contend that the case study method is unscientific because the representativeness of the single case is indeterminable. That is to say, it is impossible to establish the degree to which the single individual is representative of a collective phenomenon. Therefore, it becomes impossible to generalize the variable in question to many individuals, which nomothetists hold to be necessary for hypothetical validation. Gruhle (1928) criticizes the first-person document as created only by those individuals who are literate, excluding all illiterates and those who are less disposed to express themselves in the written word. Thomas and Znaniecki never discuss the criteria by which they chose Vladek as a representative Pole. Besides inconsistency of motive and literary ability, the sample is also unrepresentative because of the socio-psychological dynamics operating between the volunteered and the non-volunteered information. The personality structure which allows an individual to volunteer as an informant or to publicize his information is probably measurably different from that of a non-volunteer. To this criticism Allport (1947, 191) reminds the critics that their objections concerning the unrepresentativeness of single cases is true only in the nomothetic frame of reference and he clarifies the goals and methods of science:

> This conception is based upon the narrowly conventional view of what scientific method must be. Whatever contributes to a knowledge of human nature, is an admissible method to science. What does science aim to do? The answer, as we piece it together seems to be that science aims to give man an understanding, a power of prediction, a power of control, beyond that which he can achieve through his unaided common sense. Properly used, personal documents anchor a discipline in the bedrock of human experience, make the most of the predictive value of the single case in the normal process of human thought, exploit the idiographic principles of reasoning, and aid in meeting the three critical tests of

> science: understanding, prediction, and control.

Dollard (1949, 6) expands Allport's explanation, "The life-history [should be] seen as an event subject to scientific formulation and not referable to scientific canons exterior to its methods and problems."

The criteria established for methodological validation should be of the same theoretical perspective from which the case study was produced. Evaluative schemes assessing a case study's methodological validity should be created from *within* the case study's methodological context and not by extra-disciplinary evaluational schemes. This idea of not being judged by exterior standards is exemplified in other areas such as the adjudication process. The selection of jurists should take place from within the defendant's peer group and subculture, therefore judging him by standards from his own social world. This same idea holds true for academic tenure committee members who should be from the same academic discipline as the professor they are evaluating. The case study should be evaluated for its methodological validity from socio-scientific disciplines rather than by the laws of the physical sciences, which demand empirical quantification and mathematical objectivity.

The "hard-data quantifiers" believe the single case is unscientific because it fails to produce a systematic predictability scale based on measurable dimensions. Rather than rejecting and ignoring the case study by labeling it as unscientific, it can be utilized as an important scientific aid in the comprehension and understanding of scientific principles. It is often exceedingly difficult to acquire a meaningful comprehension and clear understanding of behavioral theories in sociology and psychology without some degree of acquaintance with concrete examples. Sociological and psychological theory should not be divorced from personal lives; theory is useless unless it can be related to action. It is through a case study that abstract, generalized theories in sociology and psychology are related to real life situations and human conditions. This idea of using a particular, qualitative example to understand a general principle is expounded by Allport (1947, 150):

> It has been said that a Gesetzwissenschaft employs a single case merely in order to help understand a general principle, whereas a Geschichtswissenschaft employs a general principle merely to understand a single case. In either instance, a close interdependence of *general* and *special* knowledge is implied... Not only is an initial acquaintance with particulars necessary for construction of general principles, but in the final analysis, no general principles can ever be applied except concrete and particular objects. Thus, the individual case study stands at the gateway and the terminus of specialized knowledge, and the generalized knowledge is continually being enriched by its interpenetration with what is special and concrete. In order to avoid nasty preoccupation with unnatural segments and false abstractions, psychology (and sociology) needs to concern itself with life as it is lived,

> with a significant total-process of the sort revealed in consecutive and complete life-documents. Training in concrete psychology should precede training in abstract psychology, and even the expert need repeatedly to return to the concrete life in order to prevent himself from straying into esoteric and commercial bypaths. To believe that generalized knowledge of human nature can outstrip knowledge of particular expressions of human nature is a grave blunder made not infrequently by both psychologists and by sociologists. The purpose of this excursion into the theory of knowledge is to establish the fact that "insight" is always a joint product of acquaintance with particulars (idiographic understanding) and inferential knowledge (nomothetic understanding).

The case study in this frame of reference functions as a "touchstone of reality," bringing the particularized, specific and concrete together with the generalized, abstract and theoretical. Hence, the "hard data" experimental psychologist is encouraged to form a symbiotic relationship with the "soft data" clinical psychologist, rather than the former defining the latter as unscientific and rejecting his contributions. For example, a sociologist may assign Oscar Lewis' "The Five Families of Sanchez" to field researchers prior to their entering the field to collect their quantitative data from Spanish-speaking subjects living in a barrio.

Healey (1938, 18) also stresses the instructional value of the case study:

> Students can best be taught good sociological thinking through the use of the case study method of instruction. A further value of this inductive method is that case studies of persons and family groups are of sociological value in that they frequently offer a point of view in regard to the social problems not otherwise obtainable. That only by this method can statistics and group comparisons be obtained; that case studies furnish persuasive material to secure legislation and community effort.

The case study thus functions as an invaluable and necessary didactic paradigm in the social sciences.

Induction and deduction are as interdependently related as the idiographic and nomothetic points of view. Two prominent proponents of the inductive and deductive techniques are James and Freud. James (op. cit., 32) felt that the most methodologically valid approach to the psychology of religion was through the case study and personal document. As a pluralist, James believed that no one ever perceives further into a generalization than his own knowledge of particulars extends. He fully appreciated the intensely personal nature of the religious experience and deemed that such individuality demands the idiographic/inductive approach. He found it necessary to employ personal documents authored by deeply religious individuals who described profound states of consciousness, in order to understand, "the feelings, acts and experiences of individual men in their solitude, so far as they may consider divine."

Freud also employed case studies ("The Case of Anna O," "The Rat Man," "Little Hans," and "The Psychotic Dr. Schreiber"), but unlike James, Freud is a representative of the nomothetic-deductive point of view. He utilized his cases as exemplary typifications and illustrations of theories previously formulated and not as a means of hypothetical validation. As a scientist, Freud (1933, 62) regarded the single case as a particular example of general truths:

> If we had to deal with only *one* case like that of my patient, we should turn away from it with a shrug of the shoulders. It would not occur to anyone to base a belief which has such far-reaching implications on an isolated observation, but I can assure you that this is not the only case in my experience.

This attitude, stressing reliance upon a phenomenon manifesting itself in many individuals, is upheld by many psychoanalytic investigators. Some contemporary humanistic therapists, however, are primarily interested in the unique experience of a single individual and inveigh against Freudians and neo-Freudians for their rigid insistence on Freudian classification.

In reaction to criticism from nomothetists who allege methodological anomalies, proponents of case study have initiated validating standards and evaluational criteria, thus objectifying the use of single cases. Many idiographists set out to defend their theoretical orientation by demonstrating the scientific legitimacy of the method.

Cartwright and French (1939) compared the interpretations of two independent social psychologists who analyzed a case study's data which included a diary, objective tests and subjective questionnaires, and independent oral interviews. The methodological goal of their study was to determine the degree of correlation between the reliability of predictions and similarity of conceptualization. The validity of the predictions by the two independent social psychologists exceeded their reliability; each understood correctly different aspects of the same personality. One investigator accurately predicted the subject's religious and political behavior, whereas the other correctly predicted aesthetic and interpersonal behavior. So both observers validly predicted specific facets of behavior which the critics should bear in mind when demanding observer reliability in the use of case studies.

The fact that all investigators do not unanimously agree in their conclusions does not invalidate their individual predictions and interpretations. In Stouffer's (1930) research, four judges rated 238 topical autobiographies dealing with the authors' opinions on probation. The ratings were validated by correlating them with the subjects' scores on a measured scale. The validity coefficient was 0.81. This is considerably higher than that obtained in the Cartwright and French study, but in Stouffer's study, the reliability among raters is higher still, 0.96.

The higher reliability and validity reported by Stouffer must have been due to the fact that the validity-scale focused on so narrow a field—attitudes to one topic. Stouffer (op. cit., 203) states:

> It is important to know whether inferences from life history materials can have objectivity, for it would seem that the value, even of qualitative insights, is enhanced if a number of competent observers, reading the same document, should make the same inferences. The investigation here tends to give further confidence in the objectivity of life history materials. But it should be borne in mind that agreement on inference as to a single factor abstracted from a document does not mean that investigators would agree in their appraisal of a time sequence of causal relations involving a chain of inferences or hypotheses or in their abstraction of the complex pattern of relationships.

The above statement substantiates the view that documents focused on specific topics are more nomothetically, as well as idiographically, rewarding than documents covering all aspects of an individual's life. The density of the data is relevant here, for it appears that the more particularized and topical the information, the higher the probability for agreement in validity and reliability. Hence, topical data generally yields a more reliable, valid product—on a concrete level at least, if not on the conceptual. For social scientists are more apt to agree on *what* is happening in a life, than *why* it is happening.

Baldwin (1942, 163) sought to objectify the use of "personal structure analysis." This technique, which is very similar to the method of "content analysis" was designed specifically to compensate for the lack of statistical validity within the single case. "Personal structure analysis" represents an attempt to quantify the structure of the unique single personality on the basis of a collection of personal documents. Baldwin, while analyzing an individual's personal documents (in the form of personal letters), determined the frequency with which any two classes of ideas were related in the writer's mind by employing an adaptation of the chi-square technique. From this method comes a new concept of "population" for statistics: a population of events and traits, quantifiable, within the boundaries of a single individual.

Dollard (1949, 288) responded to the nomothetists' criticism of non-objectivity by creating a scale of evaluational criteria by which validation and objectivity could be assessed during the writing of a case study. Dollard analyzed six case studies: Adler's "The Case of Miss R." (1929), Taft's "Thirty-one Contacts with a Seven Year Old Boy" (1933), Freud's "Analysis of a Phobia in a Five Year Old Boy" (1925), Thomas and Znaniecki's "Life Record of an Immigrant" (1927), Shaw's "The Jackroller" (1930), and H.G. Wells' "Experiments In Autobiography" (1934). He found Freud's case study to be the only one out of the six analyzed that met all seven of evaluational criteria and found Adler's case to meet the least. Dollard's (op. cit.,

288) educational scale is extremely useful, not only as an assessment scale for increasing the methodological validity and objectivity of case studies, but also as an outline and guide for the construction of a life-history.

Briefly summarized, the criteria are: (1) the subject must be viewed as a specimen in a culture dish; (2) organic motivation must be socially relevant, i.e., the actor's expressive and socio-physiological behavior, body language and response to internal stimuli; (3) the role of the family group in transmitting culture must be recognized; (4) the specific method of elaboration of organic materials into social behavior must be shown, i.e., the cultural and societal outlets for expression of biological drives and needs; (5) the continuous related character of experience from childhood through adulthood must be stressed; (6) the social situation must be carefully and continuously specified; (7) the life-history material itself must be organized and conceptualized.

Allport (1961, 409) attempted to improve the objectivity of single cases by devising six categories which assess the validity of the interpretations by the case study's investigator. Allport's motive for developing validating criteria is similar to Dollard's—that of objectification. Allport's criteria, however, function more to increase the validity and uniformity of conceptual interpretations and theoretical inferences. They are: (1) social agreement—if many people, especially experts, accept an explanation or conceptualization, it may be said to have presumed validity. This criterion takes on greater value if it can be shown that competent investigators have come independently to the same conceptualization. A possible extension of this test is to submit the interpretation to the subject himself for his endorsement or rejection; (2) feelings of subjective certainty—the illuminative power of a theory for the investigator who propounds (or who merely accepts) it. Though not proof of validity, this criterion cannot be discarded altogether; (3) conformity with known facts—to include known facts and to exclude none is demanded as a test for the adequacy of theories in physical science. Important though it is, it is not always easy to apply this criterion to social data (personal documents for example) where the facts are subjective and often ambiguous. But at the same time, salient events in the life cannot remain unaccounted for by any interpretation which pretends to be valid; (4) mutual experimentation—Max Weber has proposed the contemplating of the alleged cause or critical factor while attempting to imagine life without its presence. If the "experiment" succeeds, then the alleged factor is not critical. The technique of discerning causal and critical events is for the most part subjective, for it depends upon the investigator's powers of imagination: "If B had not occurred after A, would C still take place?; (5) predictive power—if an interpretation helps in making successful predictions, then the interpretation is presumably valid. This criterion is important, but it is not in itself sufficient: (a) many correct predictions are made on the basis of no theory whatsoever; (b) accurate predictions are known to be rationalized with theories that are false—as when the Greeks predicted that the sun would rise tomorrow because Apollo never failed to drive his chariot; (6) internal consistency—parts of an interpretation can be made to confront one another. Logical contradictions raise the suspicion of invalidity. True, the lines to which the interpretation apply are not themselves without contradictions and inconsistencies, but just as personality has an intricate integration wherein even the inconsistencies sometimes find a deeper resolution, so too an interpretative scheme applied to the personality has the same intricate properties of self-confrontation and congruence. No part of it should fall out of character.

Rosenzweig (1948) developed a tripartite scheme for authenticating and verifying the data of the single case by incorporating multi-measurable testing methods. They are: (1) subjective—this area includes the self-report, personal document, verbatim interview, and personality tests; (2) objective—includes ratings by the informant's acquaintance, and Q-sort tests by independent raters; (3) projective and motor expressive—includes expressive behavior (dress, gait, gestures, and facial expressions) and thematic appreciation (T.A.T., word association and picture interpretation, and Draw-a-person tests). It is certain that this eclectic gathering of information by means of standardized, codified tests significantly increases the objectivity of a single case.

Although the proponents of the case study method vigorously seek to objectify and scientifically validate methodology in the idiographic approach, the basic issue remains the same: is it methodologically valid to analyze behavior within the context of an individual life? Hirsch (1963) addresses this question of whether the results obtained with a single individual are a scientifically acceptable contribution to knowledge. Hirsch believes the methodological result to be the central question rather than whether or not the scientific method can relevantly be applied to an individual. Bolgar (1959, 31) summarizes the controversy:

> Does one single individual represent an acceptable field of study? The crux of the problem is the idiographic emphasis on precisely that aspect of the individual which is unique to him and which, therefore, cannot be explored further by replication of the same study with other individuals. Perhaps this is the same kind of controversy as the one about whether psychotherapy is an art or a science.

Allport (1961, 127) answers Bolgar's methodological question by stating that, "Whatever contributes to the systematic knowledge of human nature is an admissible method to science." And further:

> Since personal documents are, and always will be, completely subjective, there is no way of convincing the bitter-end objectivist to employ them. His demands for observer reality and public availability of the operations involved are not possible to meet. No two observers can be led to agree upon the experience and feelings reported, for there is only one observer involved. From the point of view of the objectivist therefore, there is little case to made for their use.

This methodological quandary is not so dismal as one might gather from the divergence of the opposing views. The methodological controversy concerning the idiographic-inductive approach, pitted against the nomothetic-deductive approach is often the result of an artificially produced bifurcation. As Allport (op. cit., 147) points out, "The difference between the nomothetic and idiographic interests lies largely in the coarseness and fineness of the generalization that is sought." Essentially, Allport believes that the differences between the two approaches are superficial and externally imposed. Beck (1963, 45) expresses the current position held by many social scientists in his discussion of the Rorschach method, which synthesizes two methodological commitments. He claims that the "Rorschach method both penetrates human life in its intimate reality and as a scientific tool within the framework of behavioral sciences." Hence, the two approaches *merge* through the use of an inductive empirical method utilizing objective quantifiable-deductive variables in combination with the subjective and projective responses of individuals. Other examples of this merging are found in both Murray's (1938) classic psychological study of fifty college-age men, in which he combined the individualistic-clinical approach with the statistical-experimental approach, and Thrasher's (1927) classic socio-criminological study of 1,311 gangs in which he combined direct observation, autobiographies, oral interviews, social agency and court records and newspaper accounts.

The most realistic, logical and effective stance is one which seeks the areas of agreement within each approach and combines them in a symbiotic methodological relationship. Holt (1962) argues for laying open the ghost of the controversy, claiming it is the result of "anachronistic methodological confusion." And in the final analysis, this merge of the idiographic and nomothetic approaches is unavoidable—as with the equally interdependent inductive/deductive methods, coexistence is inevitable since it is impossible to define the one without in some way defining the other.

Critics of case study method contend that in addition to the lack of objectivity due to reliance upon single cases, the case study is also methodologically invalid because of implicit and arbitrary conceptualizations. It is argued that the case study is actually more a product of the investigator's conceptual framework than a vehicle for the author's intention in producing a personal document. The theoretical orientation, academic discipline and existential frame of reference of the investigator will determine how the information will be perceived and interpreted. Going deeper into the genesis of the communication itself, an implicit conceptualization occurs when the personal document's author decides exactly what shall be said (and what shall not be said), how it shall be said, and how one shall say it. This selection process limits the boundaries and dimensions of the possible uses and interpretations of the data.

Another selective process takes place when the researcher analyzes the information. The raw data of the case study is analogous to a Thematic Apperception Test, as it is left to the perceiver (investigator) to "behold" and interpret. It is obvious that Thomas and

Znaniecki's interpretations, derived from Vladek's autobiography and other personal documents, would be significantly different from the interpretations offered by Mead, Freud, Marx, Jung or Kretschmer. One expert may see the symbolic interaction with generalized and significant others in relation to the self; another may concentrate on early childhood psychosexual fixations and Oedipus Conflict; another, the role of the proletariat in a capitalist society; another may see the collective unconscious, archetypical categories and mysticism; still another may see only the constitutional and physiological factors. Because of the arbitrary and implicit nature of conceptualizations found in the case study, critics maintain that this invalidates the conclusions and inferences obtained by this method. They should bear in mind however, that this proposed anomaly suggests that reliability is judged more important than validity of interpretation—that agreement of observations is more relevant than interpretive validity. When multiple researchers from many disciplines investigate a behavioral phenomenon, each investigator is predisposed to perceive differently, which often results in the validity of their interpretations exceeding the reliability. As in the studies by Cartwright and French (1939) and Stouffer (1930) each researcher was accurate in his predictions and yet there was no unanimity. Consequently, the case study is not methodologically invalid so long as the inferences, interpretations and predictions are correct in spite of differing conceptualizations.

The least frequently proposed anomaly holds that the case study method is invalid because no-one without a first-hand acquaintance with the particular case could understand the generalizations to their full significance. Thomas and Znaniecki (op. cit., 312) respond to this criticism, "But is it not the same in every kind of research that is dealing with concrete complexities or interconnected empirical data. That first-hand acquaintance with the data must be presupposed not only on the part of those who create the generalizations, but also on the part of those who would understand them." This alleged anomaly suggesting that comprehension of case studies is impossible without a first-hand acquaintance with the data, is misplaced, considering the fact that *no* generalized theory could be adequately understood or comprehended without *a priori* knowledge concerning the set of experiential facts (obtained through either direct or indirect means) which comprise the basic tenets of the specific theory in question.

As discussed in a previous chapter, the process of learning and comprehending is both inductive and deductive (nomothetic understanding being interdependently related to idiographic understanding). Whereas a Gesetzwissenschaft employs a single case to understand a general principle, a Geschichtswissenschaft employs a general principle to understand a single case. Both presuppose a degree of specialized and generalized knowledge. As Lazarsfeld (1940, ix) explains, "An assumption is often made that only quantitative procedures can be communicated, whereas all other procedures (insight, understanding etc.) must be left to the inspiration of the student and to the exigencies of the problem at hand. The non-quantitative methods cannot be formulated as explicitly as an arithmetical computation." This assumption fails to recognize that nomothetic-quantitative understanding is practically inconceiveable—and is also incomplete—without idiographic-qualitative understanding. When school children are learning mathematics for the first time, the teacher will invariably use apples, oranges and pennies to demonstrate quantitative processes.

In conclusion, no understanding of general laws is possible without some degree of acquaintance with particulars. The case study, however, must be clearly presented in generalized terms to avoid being so esoteric and obscure as to limit its usefulness. Cicourel (1968, 1) suggests that, "Case studies should be designed to reveal invariant properties of the social arrangements observed and interpreted. To suggest there are invariant properties discernible in case studies means the researcher must search for and demonstrate the generalizability of his findings."

## Chapter 3. Methodological Validation and Evaluation Criteria

The following is a scale by which a case study can be evaluated and assessed for its methodological validity. This scale provides both the author and the reader of a case study with an outline, or guide, which includes components necessary to render a valid portrayal of an individual's life. Together with each criterion will be a statement concerning the applicability of the exemplary case study dealt with in Chapter Four. Thus, an evaluation of the exemplary case study's methodological validity will be attained.

### 1. Comprehensive, Extensive, Historical and Chronological Presentation of Data

The case study must include a long-range global overview of the individual's life experiences. This is necessary for a valid picture of the subject's existential vacillations with changes in social position. It allows for temporal and spatial influences on the subject's personality structure and social behavior. This criterion also takes into account the fact-sheet which lists all relevant facts and events in chronological order, including everything from demographic data to significant experiences. An historical perspective is necessary to demonstrate the totality of the individual. Dollard (1949, 28) discusses the importance of this rigorous tracing of peak experiences and the interconnections of significant events which form and transform the subject's character. "Life History is a Gestalt, paralleling point by point the configurated experience of the person; in a functional sense there are no isolated parts."

(A) Case Study Model

The case study meets this criterion on many levels. First, I have known the subject since early childhood, which assures a comprehensive treatment. Second, the case study opens with a psychoanalytic section which stresses experiences of infancy, thus encouraging the subject to recollect and reconstruct his past. Third, in the appendix is a list of historical data which gives all the subject's demographic data, including family history, attitudes towards parents and siblings, aims and aspirations at different ages, sexual history, and school experience. The case study is extremely extensive in its analysis of almost every area of the subject's life. It includes not only the sequence of significant events, but also the subject's perceptions and interpretations of them: events such as parents' divorce, first sexual experience, and first drug experience.

## 2. Expressive Behavior

The thorough case study should contain a description of the subject's expressive behavior—his manner while performing instrumental actions, idiosyncratic mannerisms and gestures, vocal intonation, motoric tempo, facial expressions and handwriting. McCluhan has popularized—and commercialized—many of the information theorists' notions concerning the interrelational dynamics of technology, sensory perception, and cognitive functioning. It is upon the individual's perception that the social typification and "mapping" researcher computes data. And it is specifically the expressive components of social behavior which is perceived, identified and classified by the interviewees. In any quantitative behavioral study which explores social types, it is the expressive variable which determines the categorization of subjects on the basis of their outward appearance. Other quantitative studies not specifically researching social typification often neglect the expressive components involved in the data. For example, a drug study attempting to determine the extent to which drug-users—as opposed to non drug-users—need to manipulate their environment. What the computer would not determine (unless specifically programmed) is the amount of pressure which the subject exerts upon his/her pen when responding to the researcher's questionnaire, and exactly how the interviewees behaved during the examination.

Since every social action contains an expressive component, it is methodologically necessary for this expressive component to be discussed and interpreted when analyzing human behavior. Because expressive behavior can only be discussed on an individual basis, it is therefore the case study (which deals exclusively with the single individual) that constitutes the most methodologically valid paradigm. Hence, every case study should incorporate its subject's expressive behavior.

(A) Case Study Model

The case study model includes an entire section devoted solely to the subject's expressive behavior.

### 3. Rebuttal by Subject and Corroboration By Independent Raters

This is necessary as a means of objectifying and validating a researcher's conceptualizations and interpretations. A case study's conclusions would be methodologically incorrect and biased if the investigator did not substantiate and corroborate her/his findings through independent sources. The validity of the case study's conclusions is considerably enhanced by the incorporation into the case study itself the subject's reactions to the researcher's assumptions. This is exemplified in Freud's critique of Wittel's (1924) biography, published in an introduction to the biography proper. The responses and rebuttals by the subject to the data may function as a form of verification and substantiation of the conclusions either by his/her full endorsement, partial endorsement, or total rejection. In any case, whether the subject refutes or accepts the findings, it is methodologically important to include her/his reactions. It could be suggested that the subject has a moral right to be afforded the opportunity to react to analytical conclusions concerning his personal life.

Besides the responses of the subject himself, it is important for the case study's reliability to have conclusions based on the data interpreted and judged by independent readers. While the independent raters may disagree in their judgements, it increases the case study's methodological validity to include interpretations from a variety of sources.

(A) Case Study Model

The case study model includes the reaction of the subject, and that of the independent raters. The subject responded to the data in an oral interview (see appendix, Interpretation of Directive Interview—Tape #2) after reading the entire case study and substantiating my analytic interpretations and conclusions. When the subject does not agree with the findings, it should be noted and discussed as to its etiological significance. The case study utilized a Q-Sort Test (which describes personality characteristics) for independent rating. Unfortunately, the subject himself did not participate in this test; had he done so it would have increased the validity of the author's observations on the subject's personality structure. However, the fact that the case study was read and commented upon by the subject, and that independent sources corroborated the interpretations, demonstrates a partial inclusion of this criterion within the case study model.

### 4. Deductive and Inductive Synthesis

A case study should combine deduction and induction. This union between deductive and inductive techniques promulgates the case study's usefulness and its contribution to the social sciences. Combining the two techniques facilitates comprehension and understanding of the case study. Sperle (1933, 9) discusses this process of employing particulars and specifics in order to grasp the meanings of generalities and abstractions, "Cooley's work made it plain that the sociologist and social psychologist must start with the face-to-face, or 'primary group.' This group can be observed. The social process that is the process of interaction or of inter-adjustment among its members can be studied concretely. In a word, as a 'case study' can be made of such a group, and dogmatic theorizing is brought up against observable facts." A case study should therefore introduce its hypothetical generalized data simultaneously with its concrete factual life-story data.

(A) Case Study Model

This criterion is met throughout the entire case study. The author introduces the subject's behavioral experiences and events (often in the form of quotes from the subject) either directly preceding or directly after theoretically abstract statements. Hence, the reader is supplied with specific illustrative examples in conjunction with generalized hypotheses which constitute an appropriate balance between induction and deduction.

## 5. The Approach of This Study

Every case study should contain a statement of its author's theoretical and philosophical orientation so that objectivity may be served and validation facilitated. Perceptions, influences and interpretations are all products of one's theoretical persuasion. In this way, by expressing Freudian, Jungian, Meadian or Marxist "lenses," a reader can evaluate more objectively the author's focus on the subject.

(A) Case Study Model

I have stated my theoretical orientation in the introduction. I have also stated my philosophical beliefs with regard to the role of the case study method in the social sciences.

### 6. Use of Specific Topics

While methodologically valid case studies attempt to include all relevant areas of the subject's life to achieve a totality and Gestalt portrayal, an exemplary case study should also revolve around fundamental areas. Limiting the scope to specific topics not only increases the theoretical relevance and encourages the development of new hypotheses, but also yields a more nomothetically rewarding end-product. This is especially true when a case study has a classification index in which different aspects of the actor's life are categorized and sub-categorized under distinct topical headings. A case study therefore increases its methodological validity as well as its utility when it limits itself to analysis of fewer areas of its subject's life—rather than attempting to cover everything. Also, its utility is further enhanced if it presents its data in the form of an outline.

(A) Case Study Model

The case study model has confined itself mainly to that aspect of the subject's life which would be considered to fall within the area of non-normative behavior. It is a case study in "multiple deviance" and is therefore restricted to discussion of the subject's drug usage and sexuality. The topical theme of "multiple deviance" is limited enough in scope to qualify as meeting the demands of this criterion. In addition, the case study is divided into topical categories depicting different areas of the subject's life. This classification system is divided into two major sections—Psychoanalytic Interpretations and Sociological Interpretations—and then sub-divided into smaller areas such as the Love-Hate Pattern, Ego-Ideal, Early Traumata, Work and School Experiences, Relation with Spouse, and Self Concept. This classification system augments the topical theme and constitutes a more readily evaluated and methodologically valid product.

## 7. Interdisciplinary Approach

Case studies must be viewed on multi-dimensional levels to achieve methodological validity. If the data is not analyzed and interpreted from different conceptual reference points, it will be disproportionately biased toward its exclusive frame of reference. To compensate for one-sided conceptualizations and conclusions, a case study should include interpretations from many disciplines and perspectives.

(A) Case Study Model

The case study model incorporates this criterion by basing its methodological premise upon an interdisciplinary approach to the study of "deviance." The methodological goal of this case study model is to discover, describe, analyze and explain the subject's social "deviations" by synthesizing and compiling theories and hypotheses from a multitude of perspectives and disciplines.

## 8. Motivation and Intention of Subject and Author

A case study must state, or at least hypothesize, the motivation and intention of its subject in his/her manufacturing of the data (for example, a personal document), or in his/her willingness to be interviewed and tested. The researcher must attempt to determine and interpret the significance of this motivational factor, or combination of factors—in relation to the subject's particular area of interest, which may have stimulated the writing of the study. Even if the determination of the motivation factor is impossible, the case study's author should conjecture which would be the most probable—monetary gain, desire for immortality, emotional catharsis, social redemption or deception—or state whether the subject's production of the data was purely unintentional and unconsciously produced. The case study's author further increases the methodological validity by enclosing a statement describing her/his own motives in the production of the case study.

(A) Case Study Model

I include a statement in the introduction concerning his motivation and intentions, but fails to examine explicitly those of the subject. Although the subject's motives—a desire for psychological insight and self-awareness—are implied throughout the case study model, the fact that I never discuss them overtly renders fulfillment of this criterion merely partial.

## 9. Subjective, Projective and Objective Information

A methodologically valid case study must contain data derived from the above modes. Combining subjective information with projective and objective data validates the investigator's interpretations and conceptualizations. The author can thereby substantiate and supplement his/her inferences and conclusions by pointing to objective test results, subjective materials (personal documents) and projective materials (expressive behavior and artistic work). By combining the three modes, the case study successfully links the idiographic (i.e., subjective and projective) approach with the nomothetic. The objective tests' results are subjected to quantifiable, empirical and standardized principles.

(A) Case Study Model

The case study model encompasses all three, thus meeting this criterion. The case study contains a Word Association Test, a Draw-A-Person Test, a Q-sort evaluation, Sentence Completion Test, an MMPI, two taped interviews (directive and non-directive) and a free floating stream-of-consciousness account written by the subject while under the influence of Demerol.

## 10. Actor's Use of Weltanschauung

A case study is methodologically invalid unless it communicates to the reader the way in which the world is viewed by the subject. The subject's

Weltanschauung must be expressed and examined by the case study writer. This should include the way in which the actor views the world—his attitudes, values, superstitions, and religious beliefs. Most importantly, the case study should include the socio-psychological meaning that his existential actions hold for him at the moment of their execution. The way in which the subject perceives his own actions and their consequences should be described. The case study should use the tenets of ethnomethodology and praxeology in discovering and deciphering the rules and codes of acceptable and unacceptable conduct which operate in the subject's own social world. This is the quintessential feature of the case study method: to portray accurately the subject's world from his/her own frame of reference.

(A) Case Study Model

The case study model has established this criterion as its major methodological and theoretical goal. It fulfills this criterion by directing itself totally to the uncovering and analyzing of the subject's world view. In addition to dedicating itself to this purpose, the case study also contains a sub-section in its appendix entitled "Estimate of Self and World," and "The World's Attitudes toward the Subject" which offers a microcosmic illustration of the subject's Weltanschauung.

## 11. Family and Subculture

For methodological validity the case study requires an examination of the influences of the subject's family and subculture upon his behavior. The case study must determine the significant experiences within the context of familial relationships (or within parental-surrogate relationships) and also the significance of interpersonal relationships within the subject's primary and reference group. The researcher should analyze the spheres of influence involved in the formation of the actor's personality structure and behavioral characteristics. Familial interrelationships are profoundly important in the analysis of social deviance. Whereas Marx (1906), Mead (1928), Durkheim (1949), Merton (1964), and Parsons (1951) all discuss the societal pressures exerted upon certain individuals to engage in deviation, Goffman (1963), Dentler and Erikson (1959), Becker (1963), Coser (1962), and Klapp (1962) extend this notion of social pressure upon certain individuals to deviate to small primary group settings. It is to this perspective, where the case study is etiologically examining a subject's deviance, that the researcher must address himself. Daniels and Daniels in their paper "The Social Function of the Career Fool" (1964), and Vogel and Bell's work, "The Emotionally Disturbed Child as the Family Scapegoat" (1960), both clearly demonstrate the manner in which families institutionalize and routinize certain roles and "scripts" for specific siblings to enact. Family therapists such as Virginia Satir and R.D. Laing substantiate this notion that "social deviants" have their roles cast for them within the context of their family dynamics.

The subject's deviance must be discussed in relation to the childhood roles s/he played within her/his family and peer group. Subcultural and dominant societal mores and folkways have to be included as far as their influence upon the development of the subject's reality.

(A) Case Study Model

This criterion is met by the case study model in that it is discussed under a variety of sub-sections: "Early Childhood and Traumata," "Significant and Generalized Others," and "Family History." Under the above categories, the case study scrutinizes and investigates the role family members and primary group association play in the subject's behavior.

# Chapter 4. The Case Study

This chapter contains a socio-psychological case history of a young man who, for purposes of anonymity and confidentiality, shall be given the pseudonym of Dave. It is the central purpose of this chapter to present an etiological analysis of Dave's drug usage, homosexuality and neurosis. This analysis is essentially psychological and sociological, integrating the two disciplines for a comprehensive, extensive, interdisciplinary approach. Only through integrating the two disciplines and abstracting appropriate theories from each, can an insightful and comprehensive case history be achieved. Meaningful praxeological analysis is best obtained by viewing the subject from different disciplinary reference points. Far too often, analyses are incomplete and biased due to selective perception, whereby the analyst perceives and interprets the analysand from only one behavioral dimension. Generalizing briefly, it can be stated that sociology analyzes the existing societal arrangements, institutions, and public issues, but often ignores an individual's psychological history, personality dynamics, or self-concept, while psychology too often ignores public dimensions and public issues by localizing the problems within an individual's psyche. Any situation or circumstance in social life involves varying degrees of both psychological and sociological dimensions. Smelser and Smelser (1963, 1) describe the interdependency and interrelation of the two disciplines:

> The study of personality focuses on the individual as a system of needs, feelings, aptitudes, skills, defenses, etc; or, on one or more processes, such as the learning of skills, considered in detail. In all cases, the organizing conceptual unit is the person. The study of social systems focuses on certain relationships that emerge when two or more persons interact with one another. Thus, the units of analysis of a social system are not persons as such, but selected aspects of integration among persons, such as roles (e. g., husband, church member, citizen) and organizations (e. g., a clique, a family, a bureaucracy).... Ultimately, conceptualizations of both personality and social systems are based on inferences from a common body of behavioral data.

An interdisciplinary approach is essential to the presentation of a valid, accurate case history, for without it, functional equivalence and multicausality would not be considered.

The interdisciplinary approach recognizes and considers functionally equivalent variables, whereas the analysis which utilizes only one discipline sees behavior unidimensionally, excluding the multidimensional factors involved. The conceptual phenomenon of functional equivalence or multicausality provides a sound basis for a comprehensive, multi-dimensional case history.

For a valid meaning to be derived from a social action, it must be viewed praxeologically, from the actor's viewpoint—understanding what meaning the action held for her/him. This is facilitated by the use of an interdisciplinary approach.

Behavioral knowledge has become so fragmented and specialized that in order to attain an adequate understanding of behavior, one must be eclectic and able to synthesize new theories. This chapter eclectically synthesizes the relevant theories applicable to the subject. It does not critically evaluate the behavioral theories themselves, but demonstrates their applicability in understanding the subject's behavior.

It is exceedingly difficult to acquire a meaningful comprehension and clear understanding of behavioral theories found in the social sciences without some acquaintance with concrete examples. It is the purpose of this case study in multiple deviance to combine a real instance (in the form of a personal life) with behavioral theory.

## I. PSYCHOANALYTIC INTERPRETATIONS

### 1. Diagnostic Synthesis

Dave is the first son born to an upper-lower-class Jewish, Russian immigrant family dominated by a matriarch. The subject's father was absent during the formative years and then returned home while the subject was in the phallic stage, at which time he was acutely fixated by a "medusa head" mother (a "castrating, phallic mother"). According to psychoanalytic theory, this syndrome is characterized as follows:

(A) Early Traumata and Pathological Conditioning:

* Absence of a father as an identity figure concomitant with a seductive and over-solicitous mother.

* Mother's double-binding personality—the subject recalled tremendous inconsistencies and irregularities in his mother's giving and withdrawing of love.

* Early and frequent engagements in homosexual relations.

*Separation of parents.

(B) Personality Structure:

*Constant rumination of sexual fantasies with mother.

* Preoccupation with himself and his psyche.

* Expressed hostility toward the opposite sex.

* Much inverted hostility and aggression.

* Overt homosexuality.

* A semi-dependence on and hedonistic-escapist use of drugs.

* A deep and unrealistic need for recognition and status.

* Constant attempts to manipulate and shock others in social situations by insisting on homosexual and erotic conversation.

(C) Prevailing Environmental Situation:

Dave lives periodically with his estranged wife in an apartment near the University of California from which he has recently obtained his BA degree in Psychology. He is currently unemployed and is considering graduate school "in hopes to become a therapist

[sic]."

(D) Special Stress and Strain History:

* Promiscuity and seductiveness of mother throughout the subject's life.

* Concern about being accepted by his peers in junior and senior high school.

* Poor and inadequate sexual adjustment.

* Wife's failure to adapt to his life-style and attitudinal system.

* Concern with self-identity (especially sexual).

* Tormented by terrifying nightmares.

(E) Precipitating Event:

No one event may be considered to have precipitated this problem. However, a prior learning of the effects of marijuana allowed the subject to recognize and associate the euphoric and analgesic effects of Demerol, which in turn led to a psychological dependence on the drug. Becker (1953, 235) concludes that three fundamental steps are necessary for prolonged marijuana usage: the individual must "learn to smoke it in a way that will produce real effects; he must learn to recognize the effects and connect them with drug use; and, he must learn to enjoy the sensations he perceives." Since Dave had subsequently experienced this sequential learning process, he was predisposed to recognize and appreciate the effects of other drugs. His drug usage varied from opiate derivatives and synthetics to hallucinogenic and psychedelic drugs. The frequency of his usage is inconsistent: "I will go for weeks without turning-on, and then stay loaded for weeks." (The same is true for his homosexual activities.) Using Lindesmith's (1940) definition of opiate addiction—that addiction occurs physiologically and psychologically only when the user is able to identify and define withdrawal symptoms with the drug, and then proceeds to alleviate those symptoms with the drug—Dave is not actually addicted, but could be considered a "hard-core" user. Similarly, this marginality is reflected sexually wherein his heterosexual relations maintain his status of "bisexual" rather than that of "homosexual."

(F) Maladjustment Picture:

The subject developed psychoneurotic symptoms at the phallic stage of psychosexual development. These symptoms manifested themselves during the subject's later teens in homoerotic and autoerotic activities and fantasies. A psychological dependence on drugs developed, in which the drug's effects would provoke a feeling of verisimilitude in his fantasies. ("While I'm loaded, and making love to my wife, she really becomes my mother—or, sometimes, even *me*.") Also, the drugs were used to induce sleep when the subject was in an acute state of anxiety—witnessing hallucinatory "monsters" while hypnogogic and suffering from insomnia. The drug further mitigated passive-dependent needs, guilt feelings, frustration, hostility, and anxiety.

## 2. Gross Identifications

(A) Circumstances of the Examination:

The interviewing was done very informally: five meetings at the subject's apartment and two at my own.

They took place within a three month period, with each session lasting two to three hours.

(B) Expressive Behavior and Visualization:

Every social action contains varying degrees of behavior which are both expressive and coping. Expressive behavior is that which is non-instrumental, non-adaptive and non-purposive. The expressive content of an action is the style or manner of performing an adaptive, coping and instrumental action. It is the *how* rather than the *why*. Thus, an individual's particular and routine style or manner of performing actions would be considered his expressive behavior. Idiosyncratic gestures, mannerisms, vocal tones, motoric tempo, facial expressions, handwriting, and slips of the tongue are all expressive components.

Allport (1961, 445-461) believes expressive behavior is as equally revealing and salient as coping behavior for an adequate understanding of personality. He distinguishes between the two by stating that coping "lies closer to the level of cognitive content," while expressive:

> Is more primitive and motor: In taking a test, a subject is always coping with an assigned problem; his manner of coping with it is expressive movement .... We should put aside our usual preoccupation with content, with the intellectual, purposive, coping aspects of life, and ask ourselves what does the individual's voice, speech, facial expressions, style of clothing, handwriting, posture, gait, and pattern of gestures signify.

Strauss (1952, 22) emphasized the uniqueness of expressive behavior for an existential variation which augments Allport's definition. For Strauss, expressive motions "are variations of fundamental functions in which a person performs his being-in-the-world in a mode peculiar to him." Maslow (1954, 194) discusses the importance and relevance of expressive behavior for revealing and disclosing one's inner feelings and moods, "If a person is depressed, he is depressed all over. So, also, for loss of appetite or speech in apathy, for good muscular tone in good health, for jumpiness in the emotionally insecure person." Good health, apathy, activity, and depression are all organismic states which expressive behavior mirrors, reflects and signifies. Applying the concept of expressive behavior to Dave, it should be noted that he is tall, 24 years old, muscular and rugged-looking. His hair is light brown and wavy and he wears it parted and slightly long. His complexion is smooth and tan. Dave has light brown eyes, a long, straight nose, and thin lips. His facial expression is generally relaxed and flattened; however, when he is extremely angry and excited, his face flushes and his eyes become cold and intense. When this occurs, his appearance is very explosive, harsh and threatening. Otherwise, his posture is usually relaxed and somewhat round-shouldered, giving him a very contented, "cool" appearance. This "cool" appearance, however, is often merely a guise for an internal condition of anxiety. His "coolness" is somewhat over-determined, a compensatory reaction to internal agitation and distress. Hence it is difficult to decipher when he is actually feeling at ease and when he is being over-controlled, affecting a facade of relaxation.

Dave's dress varies from well-fashioned, expensive continental clothes to unkempt, dirty clothes, which according to him, depends upon his prevailing mood. "I usually dress the way I feel, or sometimes, I feel the way I dress—I don't always know which is the cause of which." In one sense, his dress reflects his fragmented self-concept and diffused identity, for he is an eclectic dresser—selecting his apparel from diverse styles (for example, wearing an expensive Italian silk sportscoat with dirty Levis and sandals). His sleeping pattern, too, reflects irregularity: it runs approximately from 2-4:00am to 12-2:00pm. His dressing and sleeping patterns reflect his indecision, fragmentation and attempt to play too many diversified roles simultaneously. His speech is also representative of an eclectic, ambivalent character. His syntax reveals a college-educated vocabulary mixed with slang expressions derived from the vernaculars of drug users, homosexuals, and Eastern European Jews. Dave uses first-person singular pronouns to such a high degree in his sentences that his usage illuminates his autocentric orientation. His voice is normally deep, monotonal, and quiet, but when he gets excited, it becomes harsh, and ominous. (Refer to Appendix for Personal Historical Data, Projective Test results, and transcribed interviews.)

The following quotation illustrates Dave's self-centeredness, articulateness, and grandiosity:

> I think it's my mother who hung me up the most, and that she's the cause of practically all my present problems ... I'd like to be great,

> in any sense, a god or Messiah of happiness for everyone and myself. The world is rejecting because of its own fears and because of my inherent badness ... the dope helps me to keep my head straight ... I'm closer to being crazy than most people—because I'm more aware of what's happening inside my head.

(C) Perception:

Attention was well sustained throughout all the interviews. The subject was very alert, accurate and helpful. His concentration level was intense and consistent. He volunteered information quickly and accurately. No gross perceptual distortions occurred. It was evident however, that the subject was acutely aware of every detail in the room and in the conversation.

(D) Intellection:

(1) Normal Features. (No standard test used.) According to the subject his I.Q., as tested in high school, is between 115 and 120. He possesses a fund of general information, largely inaccurate—and has a fondness for philosophical abstractions and observations. Memory was not tested, but the subject admitted to some spatial and temporal distortion and disorientation. "Sometimes I'll wake up in the late afternoon not immediately knowing where I am or how long I've slept—I miss a lot of appointments."

(2) Deficiencies. Hypophrenia is here a lack of mature mental development. Too much of the subject's psychic energy is fixated at the pre-genital stage. He therefore lacks capacity for maturation and for controlling effective and obedient behavior. This is because

because of excessive libidinal energy being dissipated in regression and immature behavior patterns. (Perhaps the "bisexual libido" theory is applicable here.) Here, fixation of a sexual impulse occurred at an early stage and that impulse was both male and female. This could be an explanation for the subject's bisexuality.

(3) Excesses. The subject over-estimates his intellect. "I'm intelligent and intellectual—over and above most people—with a potential for greatness, but it's only potential so far." Possibly, this is due to a compensatory reaction against feelings of rejection and guilt caused by society's attitudes to drugs and sexual deviance. He sees his tangential thinking and flights of fantasy as signs of genius. He has a strong desire to be different and is preoccupied with sensuality—with both pleasure and pain.

(4) Inappropriateness. Dave does not suffer from any severe distortions in judgement and is usually commonsensical. However, he has a preoccupation with taboo subjects and brings them into every conversation he can. It is his way of gaining attention. He feels he is going to be rejected and fulfills this through antisocial behavior.

(E) Thought Process:

(1) Normal Features. Thinking proceeds at a fairly normal tempo. However, at times (during Word Association Test, see Appendix), the subject's rapidity of association was hesitant. He is capable of organized, coherent, and relevant thought in relation to a goal if he is directed and not allowed to intellectualize and drift into autistic fantasies. Thinking is also marked by

loose associations and non-sequitors. He seems to strive for a stream-of-consciousness mode of thinking. The subject is handicapped by inappropriate perceptions caused by vast fluctuations in mood. This ranges from manic states to neurasthenic states. ("I get paranoid when I'm excited ... sometimes I'll wake up disoriented and afraid.")

(2) Deficiencies. In certain instances, blocking and resistance occurs, especially when discussing his childhood experiences with his father. Although during the subject's childhood his father was often absent, his father lived at home for about ten years after returning from the Service. Nevertheless, the subject cannot remember anything about his father despite being between six and sixteen during the period of his father's residence at home. When asked specifically about his father, he replies that he can't remember him at all. This may be due to feeling deserted or to a threatening and fearful memory of his father's visits home. These sudden occurrences of a masculine figure distracting his mother's love could have caused minor anxiety to the young subject's emerging masculinity. Erikson's notion of basic trust is very appropriate in understanding Dave's mistrust and insecurity. Erikson (1963, 247-248) stressed the quality of the maternal relationship as the deciding factor in the growth or otherwise of a child's ability to trust:

> The firm establishment of enduring patterns for the solution of the nuclear conflict of basic trust versus basic mistrust in mere existence is the first task of the ego, and thus,

> first of all, a task for maternal care. Mothers create a sense of trust in their children by that kind of administration which in its quality combines sensitive care of the baby's individual needs and a firm sense of personal trustworthiness. The infant's first social achievement is his becoming willing to let the mother cut off his sight without undue anxiety or rage, because she has become an inner certainty as well as outer predictability. Such consistency, continuity and sameness of experience provides a rudimentary sense of ego identity....

Thus, it is necessary that maternal consistency and predictability be present to foster trust and security. Dave's mother was very young and very immature, often venting frivolous and impulsive emotions. She probably used Dave as a husband-substitute, only to redirect her attention to Dave's father when he reappeared. Hence Dave received unpredictable, inconsistent and sporadic maternal affection, thereby producing mistrust, insecurity and a weak masculine ego identity.

(3) Excess. Dave consistently engages in intellectualization and projection. A flight of ideas can be observed in his "word chain" when he has orgasms. (Tape #2-435 in Appendix.)

(4) Inappropriateness. Dave uses autistic logic and has a tendency to modify reality in terms of his own needs. He will distort reality to gratify his unconscious desires (this tendency is dramatically displayed while

he is under the influence of a drug). People in his social world suddenly become loving and also accepting of his bisexuality. He perceives them as "having the same hang-ups as myself and everyone is bisexual." The love and affection he feels while intoxicated help eradicate the feelings of anxiety, guilt and frustration concerning his homosexual experiences. Dave is looking for a complimentary image of himself—a compromise regression to that time when he could feel omnipotent and supply his own pleasure through autoeroticism.

(F) Thought Content:

Dave is preoccupied with devising a means of controlling others. He has many fantasies involving death, coercion, violence, and blood. (Tape #2-130 in Appendix.) He also hungers after greatness and power and leadership. If he could obtain these ideals, feelings of inadequacy would certainly be alleviated. "I am a leader, not a follower. I know more than my wife about head games, and if she could get straight then things could work out."

Dave has limited ability as a clear thinker and finds it hard to be realistic and rational about his future, especially about his personal problems. His "disorder" may be viewed as serving as a sort of self-fulfilling prophecy, supplying a primary and secondary gain for him. His illness allows him to escape from forming meaningful relationships and allows him to escape his responsibility to his wife. The more he defines himself as "sick" the more he actually seems to be so. He reinforces this role by reading books on psychology and finding in them more symptoms to apply to his own case.

Dave displays weak ego boundaries and a preoccupation with interpersonal relations which he expresses in a way that is calculating, fixed and almost obsessional. The subject is obsessed with the control and manipulation of others for the love and security he lacked in childhood. The searching for his identity through a father or mother surrogate is constant. Also evident in his search for interpersonal security is his over-abstracted and unrealistic concept of others' behavior. Dave constantly compares himself with others to find similar qualities in them. He often infers these similarities (often unrealistically) between himself and another individual. "Everyone is homosexual and heterosexual—all people are actually bisexual," or "You and I have a lot in common—both suffering from a huge oedipal hang-up." Dave seeks reinforcement and "likeness" in others to inhibit his insecurities and fears. This dominant theme clearly shows obsessional tendencies, but the quality of elaboration has not yet passed the boundary of deluded thinking. Nor has it reached the bizarre level of schizophrenic thinking, and though extensive, still appears as an exaggeration of normal wish-fulfillment fantasy.

(G) Emotion:

(1) Normal features. Superficially, the affective response is appropriate and adequate. No gross pathological abnormalities exist at the moment. There are now however, underlying traits which predispose the subject to pathological behavior. He vacillates between moods of cheerfulness and optimism to those of

fatalism and deep depression. He will use drugs to perpetuate the happiness, to counteract the depression, and to control his mood swings. "I only use pot when I'm happy to begin with; if you're hung up and smoke pot, it can give you some real scary trips—it's best to smoke it when you're happy to begin with and then I go on to use something stronger (Demerol, Wyamine or tranquilizers) if I'm really uptight."

(2) Deficiencies. Although apprehension and dysphoric affect are present, these subjective experiences are largely absorbed in intellectualizing, rationalizing, and fantasizing. His conscious anxiety level is abnormally high.

(3) Excesses and Inappropriateness. Insecurity and suspicion produce Dave's deliberate aggression, as do his interest in psychology and his keen observation of people. "You can't trust people—they'll let you down sooner or later and screw you—somehow that's the way you get hurt—trusting people. You can't even trust yourself, let alone others."

(H) Action:

(1) Normal features. Dave can be quite active, persistent and energetic in certain situations, while in others, if there is too much stress and threat, he can become apathetic and self-destructive.

(2) Excesses and deficiencies. He has described days "when life seemed way too fucking harsh and loveless to get up and and go outside and face the world." He will often oversleep and sometimes spend an entire few days inside. Dave expressed a fear of going into the city because he "may be beaten up by gangs." Considering the subject's physical prowess and

fighting experience from childhood, this excessive fear seems inappropriate—not to mention indicative of poor reality testing.

Sex and violence are closely associated in his mind. Inertia, inhibition, semi-paralysis while under the influence of marijuana, as well as self-destructiveness and aggression, have all been expressed by the subject. Recently he came close to committing an aggravated assault. "It was all I could do to keep from going up and strangling that motherfucking cunt! I was so fucking irritated with that professor for not answering my questions and putting me down I could have killed him right there—I had to take six Miltowns to finally calm myself down!" He dissipates much energy in ill-defined goals and poorly chosen actions as seen above.

(3) Inappropriateness. Sexual impotence, bisexuality and autoeroticism are present.

### 3. Integrative Functioning

(A) Relations to self:

(1) Self-concept. Dave regards himself as "very intelligent and intellectual, highly endowed with a potential for greatness." He feels he is gifted with a hypersensitivity to others and thinks of himself as "psychologically honest—to the point of pain," with great aptitude for insightfulness and making others like him. This attitude masks a deep sense of insecurity and inadequacy. His unconscious feelings of inferiority underlie a negative self-concept: he fears being at the mercy of others unless he can find ways to control them. "The very first day I entered a T group I told

them that I was going to be their leader—and I was!" He is, for the most part, either unaware of his negative self-concept, or merely overcompensating by presenting an air of superiority. "I'm a great leader not a follower. I'd like to be great, a god or Messiah.... I know where it's at more than the ordinary guy."

A negative self-concept is often the product of a diffuse ego identity and of a weak sense of self. Wheelis (1958, 19) defines identity as:

> A coherent sense of self that depends upon the awareness that one's endeavors and one's life make sense; that they are meaningful in the context in which life is lived. It depends also upon stable values, and upon the conviction that one's actions and values are harmoniously related. Identity is a sense of wholeness, of integration, of knowing what is right and what is wrong and being able to choose.

Dave has consistently complained of seeing no sense or meaning in his actions and of believing that his convictions and actions are not right. His values are certainly unstable and unstructured. "Freud was right—there are unknown forces within our unconscious that determine our motivations—I'm trying to find out what they are, but meanwhile, I can't take on any meaningful changes until I get a hell of a lot more insights."

Actually, this is a superficial justification for inaction. In reality, Dave is using this rationalization to conceal his feelings of powerlessness and helplessness against the outside forces which determine his life's course. His shortcomings of judgement and decision-making are described later.

Feeling the lack of power of choice to pursue positive avenues, Dave has made the decision (or possibly a parental injunction of "Don't succeed" has made Dave's decision for him) to choose a negative identity. According to Erikson (1959, 131-132):

> The loss of a sense of identity often is expressed in a scornful and snobbish hostility toward the roles offered as proper and desirable by one's family or immediate community. Any aspect of the required role, or all parts, be it masculinity or femininity, nationality or class membership can become the main focus of the young person's disdain. Such excessive contempt for their backgrounds occurs among the oldest Anglo-Saxon and the newest Latin or Jewish families: it easily becomes a general dislike for everything American and an irrational overestimation of everything foreign. Choices of a negative identity represent, of course, a desperate attempt at regaining some mastery in a situation in which the available positive identity elements (unrealistic, unattainable material and psycho-social goals) cancel each other out. At any rate, many a late adolescent, if faced with continuing diffusion, would rather *be nobody or somebody bad, or indeed, dead—and this totally and by free choice—than be not-quite-somebody!*

Dave manifests his negative self-concept by acting out negatively defined roles. Thus, by participating in deviant activities, he gains satisfaction by perversely rejecting the previous positive and personal values.

Dave also sees himself as "cool" and as a part of the "in crowd," very liberal and broad-minded. This however, is contrary to his obsession with making others similar to himself. He has also performed criminal acts, but does not see himself as a criminal because he has always been "too smart and clever to ever get caught by the squares."

He does not view himself as a drug addict, even though he has divulged a need for and psychological dependence upon drugs. He rationalizes his drug use by viewing it as a part of his "Bohemian way of life," rather than seeing himself as an addict. Thus he has externalized the drug use, so he does not consider it a major part of his life.

The models on which Dave based his ego identity were primarily his mother and older, male, significant others. His mother was dominant in his life, and therefore, most of his self-concept and diffused identity were derived from her. His mother described him as "beautiful, perfect, flawless, her own creation, wonderful, great, and will be famous." The subject was the center of the family's attention and affection. During his identity crisis (phallic stage), his father was the object of much of the subject's hostility and aggression—the result of which was parental separation and later divorce, with the subject and his mother siding together against his father.

His father-surrogate was a science teacher who invested much time and interest in him—taking him on field trips, long walks and offering him a deep friendship. "If it hadn't been for Mr C. I really would have ended up in the lock-up—he straightened me out." The subject expressed an ulterior motive for Mr C.'s affection—Dave claimed Mr. C. was homosexual. Dave's homosexual desires and activities were further reinforced by his mother as these were less threatening to her than were his relationships with girls.

(2) Ego-ideal. Dave does not express any concrete or definite goals, other than greatness and recognition. He also fantasizes about becoming an artist with a Bohemian, counter-culture life-style. Dave's aspiration to wealth and greatness is beyond his present capacity—he has invested most of his psychic energy in his neurosis.

(3) Superego. Much of Dave's ego-identity disturbances are the result of an overbearing superego. An ego-syntonic state (vs. an ego-alien state) is only possible through a symbiotic relationship between the superego and the ego. Dave's superego is perhaps responsible for producing a major proportion of the unhappiness he feels. The basic disruptive properties within his superego are the result of inconsistent parental injunctions, such as "Be a man—don't grow up," "Succeed—don't succeed," and "Be famous—destroy yourself."

Jackson's theory (1956, 260) of the "double-bind" best describes the etiological conditioning of Dave's superego dysfunction. A double-bind occurs when a communicative gesture (verbal or non-verbal) is contradictory, containing two or more opposing messages simultaneously. Jackson offers an illuminating example of a double-binding schizophrenic mother:

> A young person who had fairly well recovered from an acute schizophrenic episode was visited in the hospital by his mother. He was glad to see her and impulsively put his arm around her shoulder, whereupon she stiffened. He withdrew his arm and she asked, "Don't you love me any more?" He blushed, and she said, "Dear, you must not be so easily embarrassed and afraid of your feelings." The patient was able to stay with her only a few minutes more, and following her departure he assaulted an aide and was put in the tubs.

Other double-binding messages are sometimes voiced, "I'm punishing you because I love you." Dave's mother often communicated inconsistent and contradictory messages regarding sex. She would sexualize her speech and non-verbal signals to Dave through double entendre, intonation and innuendo. She over-stimulated him sexually by creating and sustaining an overly intimate relationship, and then with emasculating prohibition and anti-sexual injunctions, compelled Dave to conceal his sexuality.

It is interesting to note the preponderance of male drug users who exhibit impotence, weak masculine-identity, feelings of sexual inadequacy and overly close mother-son relationships. Chein (1964, 212) found a "persistence of a narcissistic relationship with the mother—the peculiarly close relationship between the addict and his mother. It is not a closeness of warmth or mutual regard so much as it is a clinging and feeling bound together." The above is an accurate characterization of the relationship Dave describes, "She would say it's us against them and we've got to stick together."

Dave feels victimized by his mother's exploitative demands. Johnson's (1947, 1) notion of "Superego Lacunae" appropriately describes the mother-son relationship:

> Regularly, the more important parent, usually the mother, has been seen unconsciously to encourage the amoral or anti-social behavior of the child. The neurotic needs of the parent, whether of excessively dominating, dependent, or erotic character are vicariously gratified by the behavior of the child ... that the parents may find vicarious gratification of their own poorly-integrated forbidden impulses in the acting-out of the child, through their conscious or more often unconscious permissiveness or inconsistency toward the child in these spheres of behavior. The child's superego lacunae correspond to the similar defects of the parents' superego which in turn were derived from the conscious or unconscious permissiveness of their own parents.

Dave's mother came from a working-class immigrant family and married very young to "get out of the house." She is an immature, impulsive woman who uses sex to manipulate and control. She often told

Dave how unhappy and depressed she was as a child. She also divulged to Dave intimate details of her sex life with his father and relating the experiences of their honeymoon. By revealing such intimacies to Dave, she binds the relationship even closer. Dave's mother manipulates and exploits Dave to act out her unresolved conflicts. She uses his behavior as a means of gratifying her unconscious desires vicariously.

Dave's mother influenced his superego development negatively by usurping his father's position of power. Dave's father was submissive, passive and ineffectual. His relationship with his son was therefore unsatisfactory and Dave's mother became the boy's only source of security. Consequently she was viewed by Dave as both a necessity and as a threat. Being female, she was an unsuitable object for Dave's identification. The result of such a destructive triangular relationship amongst Dave and his parents—especially with his mother—is graphically described by Lederer (1964, 63):

> To be with mother often means to be a small sick boy looking out at the world from his window ("The world is just like a gigantic movie or play and I'm just watching it go by"). Sickness becomes a form of insurance against growing up ("I either feel like a very old man or a little kid") and being independent, and along with sickness, so do drinking, using drugs, flirting with homosexuality and becoming a beatnik. Sexually, the sans-identity are afraid of women. The decline of

> the father ("I couldn't even stand to spend time with him") and survival of mother ("She was omnipotent and omnipresent") may raise suspicion that mother caused father's death," that she is a spider-woman with whom one is safe as a child, but not as a man. If this view is adopted and generalized, it may lead to one of several sexual distortions: some forms of homosexuality; or, marriage to a much older woman; or, a very clearly, highly narcissistic marriage to, as it were, a copy of oneself; ("My wife is my female counterpart!") or a dependent marriage to a very rich woman ("First came her money, then I loved her").

While Dave's mother was destructive to the development of ego and superego by over-solicitousness, inconsistency and manipulative behavior, his father was destructive by default. Dave's father was detached, uninvolved and uncommitted. Dave grew to resent his father's behavior and to some extent developed what Nunberg (1955, 149) calls "a negative superego" which occurs when an individual may wish to or need to be, all that the father wasn't, for example when a person finds his own identity by opposing everything his father stands for. Dave's father exerted a polarizing influence on him which finally caused Dave to reject him outright.

(4) Love-hate pattern. Love and hate are the major axes around which the majority of Dave's interpersonal behavior revolves. Rank (1932, 80) believes that human emotional life contains one of the strongest

inner forces, and that the sex-instinct, which may be surpassed in strength by emotional life-force, can be more easily controlled when emotional life becomes insatiable. Dave has an extremely powerful need for love through recognition, assurance, and affirmation. Because of his intense introspection, he will vacillate between extremes of self-hate and self-love, consequently projecting these extremes upon others to the extent that he feels either loved and cared for, or rejected and neglected. His drug use alleviates much of the feeling of emotional deprivation and despair. Loneliness, emptiness, and anger are neutralized by anaesthetizing narcotic agents and replaced by feelings of infantile omnipotence and elevated self-esteem. Fenichel (1950, 377) emphasizes the above situation, "More important than any erogenous pleasure in drug elation ... is the extraordinary elevation in self-esteem." Dave has said, "When I am high, I feel problemless—that I'm glowing, I'm so good—confident as King Kong!"

(5) Anxiety. Of the three types of anxiety discussed by Freud—moral, object and neurotic—the latter is most relevant to Dave. Freud (1938) believed that neurotic anxiety was manifested in three distinct areas: phobic reaction, panic reaction and free-floating anxiety. Dave feels the free-floating global anxiety most acutely. He shows constant apprehension, agitation and anticipation. "I feel jumpy, like I'm waiting for Godot—always irritable and fearful, but don't know what I'm afraid of." He may well be afraid of his own libidinal impulses which he fears may filter through his ego into his environment. His id is exerting pressure upon his ego and wishes to seize control and reduce it to a state of helplessness.

Dave's life is chaotic and without organization. He is too busy with the issues of his own life to concern himself in any way with those of his "generational chain." He lacks the "courage to be as a part" (Tillich 1952, 89). Living in the present is too threatening for Dave, so viewing life as a trichotomy, he spends most psychic energy in alleviating anxiety by reliving the past or by structuring his future. Much of his drug use works to relieve anxiety. "When I get too uptight and am afraid I'll do something harsh, I blow a few joints and just relax and cool it."

(6) Insight. Although Dave is introspective, he has only a superficial insight into his problems. He views these problems as "deep-seated Freudian complexes which guide my behavior." This deterministic view fuels a fatalistic attitude toward himself. Although his technical knowledge is extensive, it is not accompanied by action, which is required if he is to solve his problems. At his current stage of intellectualization, such knowledge helps relieve some responsibility for his actions. For realistic, meaningful change, however, he must be willing to turn insight into action.

## 4. Diagnostic Summary

(A) Principal Features:

The interviews reveal an immature, deeply insecure young man who handles feelings of inadequacy and dependence by a superficially compliant, but subtly aggressive approach to people, and by an intellectual preoccupation with methods of influencing and controlling them. A dramatic example of this dual need to control not only other people but also his own intense anxiety is found in his fascination with Japanese movies about Samurai. He expressed particular delight and satisfaction over one film in which the respected master swordsman had complete control over the other characters because of his extremely long sword. Here, by identification with the master swordsman and his giant phallus, Dave indicates that he would have control and the power to destroy also, perhaps by the power of the phallus. Overt homoerotic conflict is present here and is accompanied by acute anxiety. Of all the speculative theories existing on the etiology of passive male homosexuality, Silverberg's (1952) theory seems most applicable in this case.

Dave plays a passive role with an older, aggressive partner who is usually masculine and acts as a father figure. He was fixated at the Oedipal stage having received too much sexual gratification from his oversolicitous seductive mother, who tried to make him take her husband's place. He was simultaneously deprived of love from his weak and passive father. When the subject participates in homosexual acts, he not only gains love from a father-surrogate, but also wears out this father sexually so that he will be unable to make love to his wife and Dave can possess her completely, as he did for the first five years of life.

This theory is substantiated by the subject's answer to the question, "How do you feel during a homosexual act?" "I feel like I beat him down—like I put something over on him. I feel I have to stop myself from wrestling and sort of fighting with him." It is worth noting that

Silverberg's theory works in reverse in this case. Dave's most recent sexual partner has a son near Dave's age and, according to Dave, "feels good and like he won something when I'm impotent with him." Here the partner has worn out his "son" so that he can obtain more love from his wife. Dave stated that his sexual partner was having trouble with his son, so this may be a way of evoking vicarious love as well as being a form of retaliation.

Another reasonable explanation for Dave's homosexuality could be a severe castration anxiety, which manifests itself in nightmares, suspiciousness, fear and impotence. His impotence with women ties in with his rape fantasy with his mother and his transvestite activity when very young. While passive, the subject—under the influence of drugs—can become his mother being raped by his father. His anus becomes a vagina (Tape #2-337). In this way, he avoids castration anxiety.

His obsessive introspection, projective thought patterns and expansive ideas of self are characteristic. In spite of heightened defense activity, intellectual capacity is not greatly damaged. The hyper-alertness, one manifestation of a pre-pathological condition, is in another sense an indication of ego strength which enables Dave to remain in contact with reality and to test its limits.

## II. SOCIOANALYTIC INTERPRETATIONS

### 1. Alienation, Anomie and Anomia

Dave suffers from a deep sense of global alienation which manifests itself in general feelings of meaninglessness, powerlessness, and self-estrangement. Seeman (1959) illuminates these vague feelings experienced by the subject: meaninglessness, low expectations regarding his ability to predict consequences, powerlessness, the belief that one's behavior cannot predetermine its result, and self-estrangement, the over-dependence of behavior upon anticipation of future rewards. Nettler (1957, 672) stresses normalness and purposelessness which amplify Dave's feelings about his daily life. "I don't feel a part of anything any more. The world can blow itself to hell and I couldn't care less. I guess I've got to try to put myself back into society somehow, but I keep wondering if it's worth the hassle." (It is interesting to note that the subject has recently switched his drug of choice to the psychedelic substances such as psyllocybin, mescaline, LSD, and DMT which lessen his feelings of alienation. The atarxic effects of these consciousness expanding drugs enables the subject to feel "a oneness and completeness with myself in relation to the universe. I feel I can feel at home wherever I am when I'm high." This Gemultlich, oceanic feeling he receives can be considered beneficial for it obfuscates his sense of alienation and loneliness. The subject often expresses fatalistic attitudes similar to that described in Keniston's (1965) concept of "existential pessimism " and Henry's (1963) interpretation of Camus. He feels most secure in the role of an uncommitted detached observer, not participating in or involving himself with a society which he perceives as futile and empty. Although the role offers security, its ramifications render the subject extremely isolated and unhappy. "I sit by the fountain and watch the people go by; sometimes I'm so lonely I could burst."

Keniston developed four categories of alienation: focus, replacement, mode, and agent. By using these categories, a better understanding of the subject's alienation can be obtained.

(A) Focus:

From what is the subject alienated? (1) Self. Self-alienation, as discussed by Fromm and Horney, implies a hiatus between the individual and some inner part of his being. Self-estrangement results from a lack of contact between the individual's conscious self and his inner self, manifesting itself in feelings of emptiness, unreality, and boredom. While Dave exhibits this self-alienation, he counteracts the deleterious effects by incessant over-examination and introspection, resulting in his feelings being constantly at a conscious level. Involuntary self-alienation will be discussed in a later Meadian analysis of the subject's "I-Me" dichotomy.

(2) Self to others. Srole (1956) characterizes alienation as that degree of self-to-others belongingness. Our subject feels greatly alienated and estranged from others and consequently is very dissatisfied and unhappy in his relationships, "I can't keep screwing them up by repeating the same old sick patterns." A secondary gain from his drug abuse is the "feeling of togetherness I can get at pot parties, be-ins and rock-concerts."

(3) Work and Socio-Economic Class. Daniel Bell (1959, 933), propounding a Marxist view of alienation, states that, "An individual will feel an estrangement from his 'self' by externalizing aspects of himself through the sale of his labor ... and thus, experiences a sense of distance or divorce from his society which yields to depersonalization and estrangement from work."

Marx took alienation to mean that separation and divorce of the worker from his product—the loss of control and identification with the item produced. Considering Marx's "work makes man" and Sartre's "I am what I do," it is probable that alienation from one's labor inevitably leads to alienation from one's self. The subject exhibits this alienation to a significant degree, considering that he was born and bred in a capitalist-industrial society where his work milieu has been formal and impersonal. He has thus lacked the opportunity to express his creative potential or to derive satisfaction from his labor. "I've always had to do shitty jobs, like the laboratory one I just quit—they're just a drag—boring, monotonous, and after a while, intolerable."

Meier and W. Bell (1959, 189), referring to the state of an individual rather than to a societal condition, correlate anomia with differential access to goal-achievement, "Anomia results when individuals lack access to means for the achievement of life goals," and "lack of opportunity to achieve life goals follows mainly as a result of the individual's position in the social structure." Our subject's socio-economic background is at lower class, blue-collar level. (See Appendix, Historical Background Data for details.) He feels "victimized by society," perceiving his childhood as deprived and as economically under-privileged (see Sennett and Cobb, *The Hidden Injuries of Class,* 1973 in which the authors show how such underprivileged individuals are often less confident learning new skills and are therefore less liable to participate when faced with a desirable, yet new opportunity).

There is no conclusive evidence that socio-economic class is an etiological factor in determining mental illness. There is however, a significant interrelationship between the two. Ziegler and Phillips (1961) found little correlation between symptoms and diagnoses, but did find a high correlation between diagnosis and socio-economic position.

Hollingshead and Redlich (1953) discovered significant correlation between the incidence of mental illness and social class, the incidence of psychosis being highest in the lower socio-economic range, with a lower incidence of neurosis in the upper classes. Occupying a lower status position cannot be the single etiological variable precipitating Dave's present condition, yet this factor could have acted as a predisposing variable which was aggravated by an economically depressed environment.

Merton (1964, 226) distinguishes anomie from alienation. "Anomie refers to a property of a social system, not the state of mind of this or that individual within the system—a condition of the social surroundings, not a condition of particular people. It refers to a breakdown of social standards and signifies little social cohesion."

W. Bell (op. cit., 105) distinguishes anomia from anomie by suggesting that "the former refers to the psychological state of the individual and the latter to the condition of a group or society." The subject's deep feelings of alienation and anomia were exacerbated, if not produced by an anomic social structure. The myriad of anomie-producing mechanisms (i.e., a capitalist, industrialized, competitive economic structure employing automation and cybernation; bureaucratization, specialization, and fragmentation of social and politico-economic roles; structural inequities based on race, class, and education) rendered the subject such an anomic perception that the established social mores, institutions, and structures lack legitimacy. "I no longer have any confidence or trust in the U.S.—it screws up more people than it helps." His view of himself in relation to work is diffuse and ambiguous. Becker and Strauss (1956, 253) cogently express the subject's dilemma concerning his alienated work identity, "Adult identity is largely a function of career movements within occupations and work organizations."

(B) Replacement:

What replaces the old relationship? An alienated capitalist for example may reject capitalism and adopt communism as replacement.

Dave lacks a specific replacement and remains disenchanted, detached and indifferent to society as a whole. However, his drug abuse could be considered a replacement for a paucity of involved, gratifying interpersonal relationships. He compared becoming gay to joining a club. Thus the problem of community is solved by selection of a definite, if "deviant" role.

(C) Mode:

How is the alienation manifested? An alloplastic revolutionary for instance, attempts to transform society, whereas an autoplastic psychotic attempts to transform himself.

The subject has defined ideological goals for society, but he does not actively attempt to influence the established order. His alienation manifests itself on a personal, self-involved level which causes him to feel disorganized and "not with it."

(D) Agent:

What, or who, is the agent of the alienation? The subject is outside the mainstream of society as well as apart from other people on a personal level. This alienation is too diversified and complex for us to discern when it is voluntary and when involuntary. It is circumstantial; dealing with a formal bureaucratic organization, it might be involuntary, but it is self-imposed during personal interaction. "I'm rejecting all of the relationships I have with anyone now," or, "The world is just too fucking harsh to go out into."

## 2. Roles, Reference Groups and Values

When an anomic society fails to create a sufficient number of adequate. available and accessible social roles, variance, defined as "deviance," often results.

Dave is either unable or unwilling to establish himself firmly in any existing role. His marginality between many partial roles therefore results in a diffuse identity. (Drugs are used by the subject as a means of solidifying and sustaining ill-defined role boundaries.)

Cohen (1965, 12) describes roles in relation to self as "part of the categorical system of a society, the socially recognized and meaningful categories of persons, the (different) kinds of people it is possible to become. The self is constructed of these possibilities, at some organization of these possibilities. One establishes a self by successfully claiming membership in such categories."

The subject's childhood was without any permanent or positive role model and so consequently the process of anticipatory role socialization could not develop adequately. His present roles consist of husband, student, bisexual, artist, drug user, worker and "patient." In each role, he only plays a small part; i.e., a part-time husband (sporadic separations from wife), a part-time homosexual, a part-time worker, and a part-time drug user. Therefore, not only are his roles episodic but they also lack complementarity. Thus, role conflict flourishes.

Reference groups can be divided into three general categories according to their main functions: (1) Evaluation Group—the group to which an individual compares himself for self-evaluation and self-judgement; (2) Identification Group—the group which offers the source of one's values and perspectives; and (3) Audience Group—the group by which one seeks acceptance (Turner 1956).

In the subject's own words, the people whose acceptance he seeks are "usually rich people who are not only rich, but have class—and famous eggheads, too." Economic success and intellectual ability are held in high esteem. He identifies with artists, bohemians, hippies, homosexuals and drug abusers, but evaluates himself by a comparison with successful people in business and the professions. Here, it is apparent that he has internalized a set of values which are inconsistent with his mode of living.

Cressey (1955, 116) asserts that "Behavior, attitudes, beliefs and values are not only the products but also the properties of groups." Values are acquired and maintained through individuals differentially associating with one another within their identificational reference group. Miller's (1958) six focal concerns of lower-class culture (trouble, toughness, smartness, excitement, fate and autonomy) typify the values and concepts the subject had incorporated during childhood. As he became socially mobile, his parents' values and concerns were often antithetical to those contained within his long desired social position. "When we moved from the tracts (tract homes) I became more aware of money and status—I wanted to be in with the wealthier kids and hung around their neighborhood."

### 3. Spouse

The subject states that originally he was attracted to his wife "because of her money" and later learned to like and eventually, to love her. She represented status and prestige "by letting me drive her T-Bird to school, giving her brother's best clothes to me, liquor, money, everything!" She is a very large buxom woman who appears insecure and too dependent on her husband. Her insecurity and over-dependence although sometimes burdensome for the subject, ("I've got a hard enough time keeping myself straight, let alone her head too!") allow him to feel masculine as a consequence of dominance and control. His wife takes drugs with the subject and participates in his fantasies and "games" ("We'll get loaded, regress, and play little sexual games"). And although the relationship is fragile, considering the frequent disputes and separations, the marriage serves as a stabilizer, and as a refuge for the subject. "I'd be really lost if I didn't have her to return to, to take care of me." Dependency and insecurity characterize both partners in this marriage.

### 4. The Subject's Symbolic Social Self

Mead (1913, 375) conceptualized the self as a symbolic social phenomenon arising through communication, "The self is a derivative of social life and develops only through participation (verbal and nonverbal) with the minds of others." Self arises from the individual's ability to incorporate group attitudes with significant or generalized others. Sartre (1966) defines "his" self as "my perceptions and interpretations of your perceptions and interpretations of me." In other words, "I am what I think you think of me." (This is approximately the same concept upon which Cooley formed his Mirror-Image theory.)

(A) Mead's "I-Me" Dichotomy:

Mead views the self as two bifurcated elements: an "I" and a "me," the "I" being the actor/agent which performs an action while the "me" is the observer/spectator perceiving the action. "If the 'I' speaks, the 'me' hears. If the 'I' strikes (acts), the 'me' feels the blow." Korn (1966) expands the "I" into that which the actor can do (or accomplish with a sense of control) and the "me" as that which can happen to the actor (a sense of lack of control). This is consonant with Dewey's view of experience and action as "doing" and "undergoing."

The subject's activity pattern reveals his personal interreaction as dominantly of the "undergoing" type, in which there is more reaction than action. His "me" is overexpanded during the action causing his "I" to contract. Thus, he will view himself as an object alone unto itself, feeling a helplessness and lack of control over the action ("It's being done to me—it's happening to me"). His typical activity is introjected and produces internal retroactive dialogue (between his "I" and "me") reconstructing the undergoing. This reinforces his introspection and introversion because his psychic energy is working in the "there/then" rather than in the "here/now." He feels highly self-conscious because of "me" interacting dysfunctionally with "I." His self consciousness in turn, further inhibits his ability to act; Becker (1964, 46) emphasized action in conjunction with dependency. (Refer to psychiatric report; subject's early relations with his mother.) "... the child can be undermined by considerable maternal attention or love. The natural dependency is accentuated by the mother; the child is forced to become exceptionally dependent. It is this forfeiting of the very ability to act independently that cripples his powers of 'doing' and makes him predominantly an undergoing organism." In this context, Dave's drug abuse serves as external dependency enabling him to experience "undergoing" without anxiety, while simultaneously creating a homeostatic balance between "I" and "me."

At this point Dave is best described as "drug dependent" rather than "drug addicted," although the potential for addiction is great. His drug use revolves mostly around marijuana, tranquilizers, and Demerol. Weil and Rosen (1983, 213) define addiction as, "A pattern of consumption marked by a compulsive taking of a drug, the need for increasing doses over time to maintain the same effect (tolerance) and the appearance of symptoms when the drug is stopped that disappear when it is reintroduced (withdrawal)." Dave's drug use can be characterized as "abuse," since his dosage exceeds what could be considered casual, recreational or social, but does not yet achieve the criteria required for classification as "addiction," increased tolerance and withdrawal being both absent.

(B) General and Significant Others and Self Esteem:

Becker (1962, 78) feels that self-identity, in the simplest terms is the individual's experience of mastery and control over his powers of action, and that self-esteem is a derivative of experiential actions. Since the subject's powers of action are significantly limited, his self-esteem is naturally very low, causing depression and self-destructiveness. Dave has internalized his negative and hostile feelings for his mother and father and other significant individuals. With his negative self-concept the subject seeks love and reassurance from generalized others whom he nevertheless fears will reject him. As a result of this negative self-concept, he has a limited source of sublimated symbolic modes for attaining and maintaining self-esteem. This is a tragically self-deflating cycle: self-esteem is crucial to adaptational abilities but is itself dependent entirely upon the symbolic reflected appraisals of others. Dave's sexual conflicts and drug abuse can be viewed as results of his amorphous sense of self.

Becker (1964, 104) offers a lucid and appropriate statement which demonstrates how the subject's homosexuality could be a result of his diffused self, "... homosexuality can represent a means of repleting the depleted male self—in a direct way, whereas interpersonal transactions with females can only accomplish the reverse, and this is supremely threatening to one who already feels himself empty and unmanly."

From another frame of reference, Hoffman's (1964) theories of sexuality and drug addiction are also applicable in this case. Hoffman describes the role which oedipal transition plays in the infant's development of symbolic modes for deriving his self-esteem. During Dave's oedipal transition, he did not develop the ability to switch from physiological (direct and immediate physical gratification) to symbolic modes for attaining self-esteem. The subject, not being equipped to alleviate depression (caused by a paucity of symbolic modes), came to depend upon an externalized object, the drug, which obliterated his depression. The drug intensified his orgasms and elevated his sense of self. He also had a feeling of mastery over an environment which normally consisted of a labyrinth of unattainable status symbols.

Hoffman (op. cit., 268-269) proceeds to show how a threatening, anxiety-laden object can be mastered and controlled by sexualizing it, "By sexualizing the problem, our patient transformed a distressing situation into a pleasurable one. He had no way of dealing with his feelings of envy, hostility and depression—all stemming from his sense of low self-value which was developed in relation to his brother [this applies perfectly to our subject] ... his skill in interpersonal relationships was poor: a close, long-standing relationship even with another young man was too much for him." The subject will use sex and drugs to reduce the threat to controllable size, enlarging his feelings of mastery and self-esteem. He will use "love" as a euphemism for hostility and fear of rejection. (Refer to Love-Hate Pattern in Psychoanalytic Section.) A few pages (typed by the subject while under the effects of Demerol) dramatically substantiate the above concepts (see Appendix).

**5. Deviance:**

It is my belief that no act is intrinsically "deviant." Rather, so-called "deviance" is the psychologically and culturally orientated perception of variance. The notion of "deviance," as opposed to variance, is implicitly unsavory and prompts a value-laden perception which imputes a derogatory meaning to simple difference. To label an action as deviant is to state a preference for a different specific social, cultural and ethical order. Deviation in the statistical sense simply denotes "other than normal," whereas in the social sense, deviation is used to refer to behavior which is considered bad, or at least perverse. Deviance is not created by the nature and quality of an action, but rather by the successful application of a deviant label to the action. Becker (1963, 9) defines deviance and its origins by stating, "Deviance is created by society; social groups create deviance by making the rules, whose infraction constitutes deviance, and by applying those rules to particular individuals and by labeling them as outsiders."

William Faulkner expresses this labeling process in *As I Lay Dying*, "Sometimes I ain't sho' who's got a right to say when a man is crazy and when he ain't. Sometimes I think it ain't none of us is pure crazy and ain't none of us is pure sane until the balance of us talks him that-a-way. It's like it ain't so much what a fellow does, but it's the way the majority of folks is looking at him when he does it." Merton's (1949, 275) definition correlates deviance with role expectations, "Deviance refers to conduct that departs significantly from the norms set for individuals in their societal statuses ... and must be related to the norms that are socially defined as appropriate and morally binding for individuals occupying various statuses."

By limiting the boundaries of deviance relative to the subject, "deviance" shall be operationally defined as follows: the behavior of an individual, who because of life-style, or activities, is singled out by self or others for differential treatment. Deviant action falls outside the pale of his group's concept of normal, expected and appropriate behavior. Thus, the deviant individual comes to perceive and to be perceived as "deviant."

Lemert (1967, 17) differentiates between primary and secondary deviation:

> Primary deviation is assumed to arise in a variety of social, cultural and psychological contexts and at best has only marginal implications for the psychic structure of the individual; it does not lead to symbolic reorganization at the level of self-regarding attitudes and roles. Secondary deviation is deviant behavior, or social roles based upon it, which becomes a means of defense, attack, or adaptation to the overt and covert problems created by the societal reaction to the primary deviation.

A deviation is therefore primary when its actor continues to occupy an acceptable conventional social role. "The deviations remain primary deviations, or symptomatic and situational, as long as they are rationalized or otherwise dealt with as functions of a socially acceptable role" (Lemert 1951, 75).

Some examples of primary deviations are: a businessman misrepresenting his tax returns, a housewife illegally obtaining an abortion, or a college professor experimenting unlawfully with drugs. (These are examples of negative deviation; positive deviations will be examined later.)

The subject's deviations are primary, for he acts out conventional, accepted roles (e.g., student, worker, and husband) and only engages in sporadic, episodic and compartmentalized deviant acts (e.g., drug usage and homosexual relations). His deviance is secluded and specifically located, whereas that of those engaged in secondary deviation, such as the professional embezzler, abortionist or drug addict, is pervasive and sustained.

Clinard (1963, 51) describes the possible transition from primary to secondary deviation, "Deviant action may be reacted to by arrest, imprisonment or by other sanctions. The deviant then becomes officially labeled as such and may even be socially isolated as a deviant. Consequently, he has fewer opportunities to play conventional roles and comes to incorporate a societal image of himself as deviant. When this occurs, there is secondary deviation." Primary deviation does not necessarily lead to secondary deviation, nor does secondary deviation always arise from a prior condition of primary deviation. Although most psychotics usually develop from neurotics and most heroin addicts used marijuana before the heroin addiction, not all neurotics become psychotics, and not all marijuana users become heroin addicts. Indeed, psychoses (shell shock is a common example) sometimes occur without previous neuroses, and heroin addiction (hospital addiction is a common instance) sometimes occurs without previous marijuana usage. Hence, one can remain a primary deviant indefinitely or become a secondary deviant without primary deviations. Although primary and secondary deviance are related, they are independent, so it is impossible to determine the existence of valid cause and effect. However, the generalization can be made, granting exceptions, that many primary deviations develop into secondary deviations. Dave, while presently a primary deviant, is disposed towards secondary deviance.

Stigmatization is a moral process by which individuals or groups are defined and labeled invidiously. The usual consequence is social inferiority and reduction in status. The stigmatized person possesses, "an attribute that makes him different from others in the category of persons available for him to be, and of a less desirable kind; in the extreme, a person who is quite thoroughly bad, or dangerous, or weak. He is thus reduced in our minds from a whole and usual person to a tainted one" (Goffman 1963, 3).

Stigma, in Goffman's usage, refers to a special kind of relationship between an attribute and its stereotype which can apply to the physiologically disabled as well as to the "socially handicapped" (parolees and illiterates). The stigmatization process is crucial to the establishment of a deviant identity. However, prior to discussing Dave in relation to the degree of stigmatization he is aware of (as well as to the generalized societal perception), a brief digression is necessary into the nature and elements of the stigmatizing process.

Lemert (1951, 53) summarizes the central issues:

> Mythologies, stigmas, stereotypes, patterns of exploitation, accommodation, segregation and methods of control spring up and crystallize in the interaction between the deviants and the rest of society. The informal, societal reaction

> is extended and formalized in the routinized procedures of agents and agencies delegated with direct responsibility for penalizing and restraining or reforming the deviants. The status of the deviants is redefined and special pariah roles may be assigned to them.

The ironic, self-defeating tragedy which occurred during medieval England's public degradation ceremonies (more pockets were picked during public executions than on any other day) is still operating in the form of the contemporary stigmatization processes. The very agents and agencies invested with responsibility for penalizing, restricting or reforming deviants, in fact, often create and maintain deviance through stigmatizing individuals. These labeling and defining agencies (criminal courts, departments of correction, probation and parole, and psychiatric clinics) promulgate and perpetuate the very situations and conditions they attempt to reduce. Ironically, the efforts aimed at containing specific behavior often make it proliferate instead. Matza's (1964) discussion of the etiology of juvenile delinquency illustrates this self-fulfilling deviant prophecy. Matza begins his description of the process by placing the juvenile in a state of drift between convention and crime. The youth exists in an "adolescent vacuum," a condition for which society has failed to provide available, accessible and appropriate definitional roles. Thus, he feels powerless, tentatively acting out ill-defined roles. All learning behavior involves an initial "acting-as-if" stage before "becoming." The youth seeks a role in which he can formulate and establish an identity and simultaneously associates with a delinquent sub-culture which in turn identifies with criminal role models. At the point where apprehension and adjudication occur, his marginal "acting-as-if" role becomes solidified and sustained.

The entire adjudication process can be viewed as a "dramatization of evil" in which criminal self concepts are created through stigmatization, and primary deviance is transformed into secondary deviance.

In a parallel discussion, Wilkins' (1964) feedback model indicates the role of stigma in the creation of deviance, "Less tolerance leads to more acts being defined as crimes, which leads to more action against individuals; which leads to more individuals perceived, labeled and defined as deviant; which leads to more deviant and criminal self-conceptions; which leads to alienation and exclusion of deviants; which leads to more crimes by deviants; which leads to less tolerance of deviants by conforming groups; which leads finally to more acts being defined as crimes. Thus, stigmatization is not only a result, but also a cause of deviance.

An identity which is deviant through stigmatization has not yet been established in the subject to any significant degree because he has not been apprehended and labeled by law enforcement authorities. His deviations give rise to the potential establishment of a deviant identity through the possibility of detection, apprehension and prosecution. The subject, however, considers himself something of a pariah with a sense of victimization and exploitation—psychologically by his mother, and economically, by society. On the scale below, which classifies deviation and the degree of stigmatization attached to it, the subject would appear between level C and level D.

DEVIATION: A1, B1, C1, D1.

STIGMATIZATION: A2, B2, C2, D2.

(A1) No deviation; (A2) No stigmatization; (B1) Situational deviation. A deviant action which is a direct spontaneous response to an appropriate external event—death of a loved one, disaster, and disfigurement. Here the nature of the situation determines the appropriate boundaries of the deviant response; (B2) Stigmatization. The degree can vary from low to high depending upon the nature of the external event, and upon the the degree of morel turpitude attached to the actor's response; (C1) Primary deviation. The deviation is not symbolically internalized into dominant self-conceptualization and is integrated into the socially acceptable role; (C2) Stigmatization. There is little or none due to lack of negative appraisals from others; (D1) Secondary or Professional Deviation. The deviancy is incorporated and internalized so that the actor derives major ego satisfaction as well as economic gain; (D2) Stigmatization. The highest degree, due to the actor's frequent encounters with defining authorities and self-defined deviant career.

Goffman identifies two distinct groups of stigmatized individuals, the *discreditable*, and the *discredited*. The former includes those who assume that the activity for which they are stigmatized (drug abuse, homosexuality, unemployment, and political activism), is not immediately perceivable by others; the latter term refers to stigmatized individuals who assume immediate perception of that for which they are stigmatized (physical deformity, speech defect, or membership of an ethnic minority). The degree to which a person feels stigmatized is indicated by the coping mechanism utilized to deal with the stigma. Rationalization, justification, excuse and denial are various means frequently employed in coping with a stigmatized self. The subject often rationalizes his homosexual activities, "All people are basically bisexual anyway," and "I may fool around, cavort and pervert a little, but I'm not a faggot." The latter statement is indicative of a phenomenon discussed by Reiss (1961, 108) who shows how enterprising juveniles deal with economically-based homosexual activities by simultaneously accepting and rejecting portions of the stigma. The subject rejects a total homosexual stigma by reducing it to "bisexual experiences."

The rationalizations concerning Dave's drug abuse are similar to those employed with respect to his homosexual activities. "I get loaded when I'm uptight and want to relax sometimes, pretty often when I'm depressed, but I'll *never* become a strung-out, stoned-cold junkie."

His drug abuse and homosexual activities are felt to be *discreditable,* but he is not *discredited.* The subject feels "stigmatizable," yet not actually stigmatized, because he has control over whether or not to conceal or reveal his deviations. His prerogatives and freedom of choice in this matter certainly mitigate the stigma associated with his deviations.

Deviations can be justified and/or excused—Lyman and Scott (1957, 2) define justification as "an act in which the actor accepts the responsibility for his action, but denies the pejorative quality associated with it." Matza (1964, 41) states that justification, "asserts the righteousness of an act in and of itself. A wide assortment of behavior has been justified in this way, ranging from the radical homosexual's assertion that love between men is an indication of higher sensitivity, to the assassin's belief in the righteousness of regicide."

H. Becker (1963, 3) shows how those who fail to conform to a group's rule are labeled "outsiders" and use justification in coping with their deviant behavior, "Some deviants (homosexuals and drug addicts are good examples) develop full-blown ideologies explaining why they are right and why those who disapprove and punish them are wrong." Excuses are simply acknowledgements of guilt, yet in the process of excusing, some responsibility is relieved because an external element—a person or a thing—is held partly or fully responsible.

The subject will vacillate between excusing and justifying his deviations. The salient determining variables are the particular deviation, the deviation's temporal and spatial dimensions, and the nature of his audience.

If he is at a "straight" party, and he has participated in a homosexual act in an automobile just prior to entering the party, he would be more apt to justify his action than to excuse it. If casually talking to a professor in a detached, intellectualized manner concerning his drug use, he may excuse it. "My mother is really sick, I'm certain it was her who hung me up so badly—I have to use drugs to relax and sleep." Or something of that nature.

There is a strict separation in his selection of deviant partners. He will select partners for homosexual activity (e.g., professors) from outside his peer group but will look to his peers and contemporaries as partners in drug abuse. Bieber's (1962, 114) discussion of homosexual mate-choices suggests an explanation for the subject's choice of non-peer group homosexual partners:

> A detached pattern of father-son relatedness obviously promotes a defective relationship to which the child may react multifariously. He may develop a cognitive awareness of a lack of paternal affection, warmth and interest, or he may be unable to formulate the lack and may merely experience a vague hunger or yearning for something he cannot identify. Some children may interpret detachment as rejection, but in any case, no matter how it is experienced, it is always traumatic. The child may attempt a way out by seeking other reparative relationships to fulfill his yearnings—often with other males. Thus, the pathologic seeking of need-fulfillment from men has a clear point of origin in fathers who were detached.

The subject does not frequent commercialized homosexual settings such as bars, night clubs, or baths, but encounters partners spontaneously and in conventional social settings. On the other hand, the subject frequents commercialized establishments to obtain drugs. He will purchase drugs from professional dealers and often spend his evenings at all-night restaurants where drugs may be purchased, and go to drug parties and "shooting galleries." (The subject's parental history—an exploitative mother and detached, aloof father—has been discussed in a previous section.)

The subject made an astute general observation while commenting on his affiliations and predisposition towards drug use, "Catholics and Protestants use lush (alcohol), Jews use soft drugs (marijuana, amphetamines, barbiturates and psychedelics), bikers like to shoot speed (inject methamphetamine), and blacks shoot hard stuff (heroin)."

Perhaps deviance is sub-culturally defined and determined by functionally equivalent modalities of expression. In the subject's sub-culture, using "soft drugs" was one of the modes defined and employed for deviant and rebellious expression. (It is interesting to note the W.H.O. assertion that one-third of the people presently acting out a deviant role through drug abuse would stop doing so if narcotic abuse were re-defined as non-deviant activity.)

In considering the subject's affinity and predisposition towards the selection of a deviant role, an enlightening description of this selection process is found in Wilkins' (1967) informational model. Wilkins theorizes the components which lead to rational decision-making. According to Wilkins, there is a direct proportionality between meaning and predictability; for something to be meaningful, it must be predictable. Predictability is dependent upon information; information is operationally defined as that which reduces uncertainty. Information must be abundant, available and accurate to facilitate rational decisions. For successful decisions, it is necessary that symbolic modes for attaining information are developed.

The subject's conflicting mental states will often obfuscate his perception which in turn, alters the information upon which he bases his decisions. (Refer to socio-psychological modes for attaining and maintaining self-esteem through the reflected appraisals of generalized and significant others—found in the previous section on the subject's Symbolic Social Self.) The subject states, "People are always playing their little games ... trying to put you down—you can get hurt if you listen to what people are *really* saying," and "Sometimes I feel so helpless and insecure, I get so lethargic, it's impossible for me to function."

Abercrombie's (1960, 41) analysis of judgement emphasizes the subject's difficulties in decision-making through his poor assimilation of information. "The mentally sick are those whose store of information is inappropriately organized; their schemata or assumptions are such that the information they receive from the environment, both physical and social, does not lead to effective action." It has been suggested that schizophrenia is the "quintessence of indecision." The subject's difficulties in making decisions are manifested in his recurring feelings of helplessness, powerlessness and lack of control. His deviations often are ramifications of indecision rather than premeditated judgement, or they are results of hasty, regretted decisions (based on misinformation) for which he later feels tremendously guilty. "Lots of times, I'll get loaded when I really didn't want to ... It (the drug) was just there," and "I won't set out looking for sex, it seems 'it' finds me."

The subject's psychic and social predisposition towards deviation is amplified by the disproportional number of deviant outlets provided by his environment. The San Francisco Bay Area offers abundant opportunities for drug abuse and homosexual activity.

Until recently, deviance was viewed from a reformist angle. This meant deviations were regarded as negative and dysfunctional and required the reduction and elimination of deviance. The naturalistic approach, which gradually replaced the reformist throughout the sixties and seventies, attempted to view deviations praxeologically and descriptively, without prescriptive value judgements; to see the deviant from his or her referent point, and capture objectively his or her lifestyle, values, and orientation. Throughout the last seven or eight years however, this enlightened attitude has suffered serious setback and recently, the reformist approach has re-emerged as dominant.

Despite the fact that many insightful social thinkers such as Durkheim, Marx, Mead, Parsons and later Dentler, Dubin and Coser, stressed the functional necessity of deviance, the reformist approach ignores these functional elements. They found that deviance plays a key role in social change and advancement, unifying various groups and solidifying their cohesiveness, differentiating and defining other groups and their moral and ethical codes, maintaining society's psychic equilibrium and organizational efficiency.

Dubin emphasized the innovative quality of deviance in relation to social change (1959, 47-64). Similarly, Parsons found deviance a major role in the origin of change within a social system (1951, 250). The Aristotelian notion of truth (truth lies between two extremes, with deviations extending the extremities) dialectically manifests societal change. Decision-making is enhanced by increased information fed back into the system through deviation. Deviations also function for societies and organizations by providing "warning signals" through dissent, disturbances and defections. Hence, valuable information is supplied by deviance which aids in decision-making.

Automation and cybernetics, used as analogues, demonstrate this contribution of deviance for societal change. Automation is static, deterministic and anti-variant, while cybernetics is dynamic and continually self-optimizing through variation.

Social groups can acquire cohesiveness and solidarity by uniting themselves either against or on behalf of the deviant. Coser (1966, 9) remarks that:

> Nothing unites the members of a group like a common enemy. Competition for wealth, power, status and other values, divergent philosophies, boredom, frustration and fatigue—all these drive people apart, undermine morale

> and impair the efficiency of the group. An external enemy who threatens or is believed to threaten what the members of the group cherish in common, arouses the sentiments of the community and revives a waning solidarity.

Mead's (1928, 9) example of the criminal typifies this function of the deviant:

> The attitude of hostility toward the lawbreaker has the unique advantage of uniting all members of a community in the emotional solidarity of aggression.... The criminal does not seriously endanger the structure of society by his destructive activities, and, on the other hand, he is responsible for a sense of solidarity, aroused among those whose attention would otherwise be centered upon interests quite divergent from those of each other.

When a member of a family, club or organization deviates, the result often leads to a unified demonstration of protection, kindness and assistance by the group on behalf of the deviant member. Neighborhood members become unified when attempting to reduce juvenile delinquency by establishing Boys' clubs, athletic leagues, or half-way houses.

The philosopher Leibniz noted that one could not appreciate the sweet without previously experiencing the bitter, and Shakespeare noted that "the good deed shines brightest in an evil world." And Durkheim pointed out that, "in a community of saints, there would be at least one sinner to define what is saintly." Deviation provides the *contrast* necessary for accentuating conformity. Thus conformity becomes desirable and creates a sense of community among conforming individuals. A group's "three Rs" (rules, regulations and restrictions) are clarified by deviations; the boundaries of acceptable behavior are clarified.

Deviance is also necessary to maintain society's psychic equilibrium and homeostatic balance. Conforming members of society are able to watch their unconscious (and conscious) desires acted out for them via the mass media—by deviants. Thus, by vicariously experiencing and satisfying deviant wishes and desires, deviant *actions* are averted.

Durkheim (1949, 99-103) felt that, "social structures exert a definite pressure upon certain persons in society to engage in non-conforming conduct." Mead's (1928, 577) contention corroborates Durkheim's theory, that a system of deterrent punishments not only fails to repress crime, but also "preserves a criminal class." The law enforcement policies and procedures governing prostitution, pornography, gambling and drug sales illustrate this point. There is also a secondary gain derived in prosecuting the individuals involved in providing avenues for deviation: guilt is diminished by a purification process achieved by punishing the offender. Thus, many deviations are produced, promulgated and perpetuated by society to serve as a necessary "outlet" for society's stability and general well-being.

Organizations and bureaucracies would be inefficient and ineffective without operationalizing varying degrees of deviance into their systems. Deviance becomes one of the central operational devices which sustains the organization or bureaucracy, and is often informally institutionalized as a permanent procedural aspect. Gerver and Bensamen (1964) analyzed crimes and punishments within an aircraft factory and found that illegal shortcuts were condoned by foremen and inspectors. They also found that the deviations incorporated into daily work were only ceremonially dealt with when discovered.

In England, when organizations (e.g., post office, railroad, and other essential services) are forbidden by law to strike, dissatisfied workers express their dissatisfaction by implementing an opposite form of strike known as "working to rule." This entails the *strictest* adherence to the organization's rules *without any deviations.* The obvious result (inefficiency) magnifies the necessity of deviance to the vitality and success of social systems.

The functions and dysfunctions of deviance must be simultaneously considered from two frames of reference, that of society and that of the individual. One of the Taoist maxims dictates that in every action there exists both good and evil. Therefore, inherent within each deviation there is both a function as well as a dysfunction.

The subject's sexual deviations serve him in much the same way that prostitution serves society, according to Davis' (1937, 774-759) description of prostitution, by providing a necessary sexual outlet. For the subject, the outlet is needed so that he might avoid threatening heterosexual relationships. Lemert (1967, 48) describes a positive aspect of homosexual deviation:

> Becoming an admitted homosexual (coming out) may endanger one's livelihood or professional career, but it also absolves the individual of failure to assume the heavy responsibilities of marriage and parenthood, and it is a ready way of fending off painful involvements in heterosexual affairs.

Dave is thus able, through homosexual affairs, to answer his sexual needs, gain parental love from a father-surrogate, and to avoid heterosexual commitments and responsibilities.

His deviations with drug abuse also serve as a necessary outlet for reducing psychological stress and conflict. A secondary functional aspect of his drug abuse lies in the enhancement of his creative talent. The subject feels that his art (paintings and sculptures) has improved as a direct result of drug-induced experiences.

It has been said that morphine reduces the murderer to a mere thief. In such a case, the morphine would operate to reduce the severity of the deviation and therefore act in a manner analogous to the defense mechanism of the psychiatrist's patient. In both cases, before abstracting either the drug or the defense mechanism, extreme care must be taken to insure that a functional equivalent is provided to inhibit the emergence of a deviation of greater magnitude. The subject's deviations function for him by reducing intolerable situations and circumstances to bearable size.

**6. Diagnostic Impression**

Rather than diagnosing the subject in the classical vernacular of the psychopathological categories, I believe that a more accurate diagnosis is achieved by utilizing Menninger's (1963, 162-212) Five Levels of Deviations and Disruptions nosology.

Menninger holds that far too often individuals are labeled, defined and classified into meaningless psychopathological categories which usually amount to nothing more sophisticated than certified "name-calling." On Menninger's scale, which is stratified by degree, deviation and departure from the mean, the subject vacillates between levels one and two:

> 1) The first level or stage or degree of departure from the normal is that state of external and internal affairs which in common parlance is usually called "nervousness." It is a slight but definite impairment of smooth adaptive control, a slight but definite disturbance in organization, a slight but definite failure in coping and frequently characterized by hyperkinesis (extreme restlessness and overactivity), hypersuppression (a conscious effort in self-control), hypervigilance (exaggerated perception) hyperintellection (worry), hypercompensation (denial) and/or somatic reactions (minor somatic and sexual dysfunctions). 2) A second level or stage or degree of departure from the formal level to increased disorganization is one which in normal life rarely results in resignation or hospitalization: it is that

group of syndromes which harnesses individuals to the necessity for expensive compensatory living devices. These are painful symptoms and sometimes pain those looking on as much as the patient. In the last half-century they have been called "neuroses" and "neurotic syndrome," but these are not good names. The syndromes are thousands of years old.... Prominent in all second level departures is the presence of subjective discomfort. It may be vague or it may be specific. It may be uneasiness or anxiety—a mild depression, a sense of things as not being right or comfortable or pleasant. This is persistent and sometimes almost frightening. *More often however, there is a chronic gnawing sense of failure, of uselessness and incompetence, of being a great disappointment to oneself and to others.* Second level disorders are: A) Aggressive discharge blocked from consciousness by dissociative withdrawal: 1) Phobias and counter-phobic states; B) Aggressive discharge displaced to the body: 1) Self mutilation, 2) Somatization (in fantasy, function and structural impairment), 3) Intoxication and narcoticization; C) Aggressive discharge effected though symbolic and magical modifications: 1) Perverse sexual modalities, 2) Addictive personalities, 3) Our third stage of regression or dysorganization or disequalibrium or dyscontrol, is characterized by the escape of the dangerous destructive impulses, the control of which has caused the ego so much trouble. These are the outbursts, the attack, the assaults and the social offenses which result from a considerable degree of ego failure, 4) A fourth order of dyscontrol involves still more ego failure. Reality loyalty is almost completely abandoned; there is disruption of orderly thought as well as of behavior; there is demoralization and there is confusion. These are the classical pictures of medieval psychiatry, the "lunacies" of our great-grandfathers, the "insanity" of our grandfathers, the "psychoses" of our fathers, 5) A fifth and penultimate stage is proposed (an extremity beyond psychoses in its obsolescent sense), *the abandonment of the will to live.*

Menninger's third category best describes the stage or level of dysequilibrium and deviation the subject could enter and act out, given enough stress. Presently, he remains in between levels one and two. Determining the majority of Dave's behavior is the self-defeating, self-destructive, success/failure dichotomy found in the heroes of classical tragedy. It is a central feature of tragic heroes, as described by Aristotle in his *Poetics,* that the hero is both active and conscious in his self-destruction.

This tragic flaw, hamartia, is inherent in all tragic heroes. The hamartic component in the subject is similar to the success/failure theme in the myth of Icarus. According to the myth, Icarus desired too much and, in his unreasonable strivings, flew too near the sun and ended his life tragically after soaring to forbidden heights. Many other myths portray this tragic theme: Sisyphus forever pushes a boulder up a hill only to have it roll back down every time he reaches the top; Erostratus, in seeking eternal fame became a criminal by burning down one of the seven wonders of the world, the Temple at Ephesus; Prometheus, having illicitly brought the heavenly fire to earth is condemned to a millennium of being eaten alive; and Tantalus, having stolen the ambrosia of the gods, suffers a fate that makes his name a symbol of an exquisite form of torture. The tragic flaw possessed by the subject is also similar to that of Hamlet, whose indecisive "To be or not to be" caused him much anguish. The subject uses indecision, non-involvement and non-commitment to avert even the possibility of failure. The subject is saying, "To decide or not to decide...? As long as I don't decide, I may not succeed, but I certainly cannot fail." His indecisiveness prohibits involvement, participation and commitment. The subject feels safer remaining in a vague, ambiguous, innocuous position. However, the indecisiveness itself is a form of failure for it is unproductive, ineffectual and a self-defeating defense mechanism.

The etiological base for the subject's dyscontrol, dysfunction and deviation is an "Icarus-Oedipus Complex" in which the subject's unresolved oedipal complex dictates impossible demands. The subject's dominating, overly-controlling mother fostered an excessively intimate relationship which resulted in a fixation of his psychic energy in the oedipal stage of psychosexual development. The subject internalized his mother's unrealistic expectations concerning financial success. He desires tremendous wealth, "So I can feel economically and psychologically independent from everyone." The subject's wishes for affluence and opulence are unrealistic and unattainable, at least by legitimate means, in his present condition.

### 7. Prognostic Indications

At the present time, the subject needs the ramifications of his "mental illness" for its secondary gains. His "psychological problems" perceived as an illness, release him from the reponsibilities, commitments and involvements which threaten him in the maintenance of a successful marriage, the sustaining of gainful employment, participation in the positive, productive and self-fulfilling activities of human society.

He expressed this need to be perceived and to perceive himself as being "mentally ill" by discontinuing psychotherapy when it was disclosed to him that he was not as "ill" as he had thought or as he would like to be.

He perpetuates and reinforces his "illness" by masochistically applying to himself pathological symptoms and acting out destructive deviations.

I foresee three possible alternative prognoses for the subject: (1) He may become addicted to drugs (perhaps with all of his problems becoming focused on one real crisis, instead of the global anxiety he now suffers), he will accept the role of "patient," undergo a real surrender, and work through a "rebirth process"; (2) He may seek psychotherapeutic help again and, with the aid of a professional, gain important insights and overcome much of his self destructive behavior; (3)

He may commit a sexual crime involving violence, or he may be apprehended for illegal possession of drugs.

# Chapter 5. Conclusion

Prior to any analysis concerning the methodological validity of the case study paradigm as employed within the social sciences, a clarification and amplification of the means and goals of social science is necessary.

The means and goals of the social and behavioral sciences should be discussed in relation to methodologically popular and academically fashionable trends which currently influence ideologies. I believe that *understanding,* and not dissecting, categorizing and classifying, is the true goal of the social sciences. Perhaps in the social sciences, the zeal to compete with the mathematical objectivity and empirical quantification demanded by the physical sciences has resulted in the theoretical goal being obfuscated by the means. The rigorous scientific rubrics of physical science coupled with the advent of electronic data processing may have resulted in a preoccupation with methodological means and an overemphasis on the nomothetic approach, while concomitantly underestimating the idiographic approach to understanding human behavior. The idiographists and naturalists feel that their experimentally (nomothetically) oriented colleagues may have become overdetermined in their quest for empirical means and methodological quantification. The Mertonian adaptation scheme of the ritualist probably most accurately describes the idiographists' complaint: an individual overstressing the means tends to lose sight of the ends. "Hard-data" quantifiers often tend to place too much importance upon the acquisition of measurable and observable facts which objectify knowledge while placing too little importance upon subjective non-quantifiable, experiential understanding. Cooley's (1926, 59) investigation into "The Roots of Social Knowledge" produced a dichotomized view of the genesis of knowledge:

> Approaching the study of Knowledge from the standpoint of its evolutionary genesis we find that there are two distinct sorts, which may be called spatial and social. The former, based on sense perceptions gives rise to exact or measurative science. The latter, based on the "mental-social complex" gives rise to a sort of knowledge essentially sympathetic or dramatic which is lacking in that exact agreement upon elementary perceptions which is necessary to true measuration. Statistics is a method of manipulation, not of perception. Interpretation and prevision in sociology as in other sciences, is a work of the constructive imagination.

Here, Cooley's term "Social Knowledge," which connotes non-empirical observations from subjective consciousness, is synonymous with the term "understanding." This distinction between knowledge and understanding is illuminated by Aldous Huxley (1956, 32):

> Knowledge is acquired when we succeed in fitting a new experience into the system of concepts based upon our old experiences. The old is our home-made system of ideas and word patterns. It is the stock of finished

> articles fabricated out of the given mystery by memory and analytic reasoning, by habit and automatic associations of accepted notions. Knowledge is primarily a knowledge of these finished articles. Understanding is primarily direct awareness of the raw material. Understanding comes when we liberate ourselves from the old and so make possible a direct, unmediated contact with the new, the mystery of our existence.

What Huxley is saying is closely connected to what Zen Buddhists mean when they state they have reached Satori, the Buddhist state of consciousness which has been described as "seeing the world with new eyes." One achieves the psychic state of Satori when one has successfully transcended their ego-boundaries and loses their sense of self into another realm of reality. Understanding is the product of illumination via a form of a transcendental experience. Gendlin (1962) describes the experiential "felt-meaning" of idiographic understanding by the process of intersubjectivity or entering another's socio-psychological category. Skolnick (1966, 41) followed this premise in his case study methodology. "In attempting to understand a social or political process such as democracy, oligarchy, bureaucracy, or justice, the process itself must be learned in intimate detail. To do this the researcher must immerse himself in it."

Peter Demianovich Uspenskii attempted to control his consciousness so thoroughly that, while under the influence of a consciousness-expanding drug, he could still retain enough control to record an explanation of that feeling of revelation and illumination which is left in the memory after the effects of the drug wear off. He wanted to control the profound psychedelic experience of consciousness expansion. After preparing the pencil and paper to document his experiences and explanations, and ingesting the drug, he fell into an ataraxic-euphoric state. He made one futile attempt to write and then lost consciousness. Hours later when he regained consciousness, he wrote four words: *think in other categories*.

Philip Wylie (1942, xv) wrote:

> To physicists, chemists, biologists, medical doctors, sociologists, economists, Columbia professors and all other such mechanics, thinking in other categories, is, in solemn truth, a most profound challenge. They are so busy promulgating the marvels they have uncovered in the single category with which they concern themselves that they never admit the possibility of another. They do not want incomprehensible competition.

Carl Orff, the contemporary composer, has refused to accept as a student anyone but the pre-school child—the child whose spontaneous sensory perceptions have not yet been channeled by biased literary and visual categories.

The case study paradigm facilitates understanding by offering categories which would otherwise be unapproachable. Berger (1963, 4) defines sociology "as an attempt to understand." Case studies offer social worlds for one to enter and leave with understanding. Weber emphasized subjectivity and asserted that sociological understanding—Verstehen—is impossible without consideration of the entire subjective dimension of human behavior. Allport (1947, 149) delineates the goals of scientific methodology by asking:

> What does science aim to do? The answer as we piece it together from the writings of many authorities, seems to be that science aims to give man an understanding, a power of prediction, and a power of control, beyond that which he can achieve through his own unaided common sense. If we abolish preconceptions as to what the scientific method *must* be, and fix firmly in mind this threefold *goal* of science, we conclude that the study of personal documents unquestionably has its place in science. It is unfortunate that recent discussions of scientific method have produced a ritualism that seems to say the language of science is more important than its purposes. Our position, on the contrary, is that if the language of personal documents can be shown to enhance understanding to confer powers of prediction and control, then the use of these documents must be admitted as valid scientific method.

If one of the central goals of social science is to understand human behavior, then it is reasonable to conclude that any paradigm that contributes to the systematic body of knowledge concerned with human behavior is an acceptable and valid method. The case study contributes to an idiographic understanding of human behavior and therefore should qualify as a methodologically valid paradigm in the social sciences. The case study is particularly methodologically valid when it is evaluated and assessed by criteria formulated within its own ideological frame of reference. As pointed out earlier, standards of judgement should be developed within the relevant area (i. e., a judicial board's members should be within the defendant's peer group) and not from an exterior referent point. The case study must incorporate its own evaluational and assessment criteria and include measurable validational and verificational codes designed for its particular methodological problems. Schemes for determination of methodological anomalies, invalidities, and deficiencies should be the products of the same theoretical orientation from which the case study was created.

Stating that the case study is a methodologically valid paradigm does in no way discount, discredit or reject other methodological approaches. On the contrary, this statement merely suggests that more emphasis and stress should be placed on idiographic approaches in social science. This statement does *not* mean to imply the exclusive use of the idiographic approach or to invalidate the nomothetic approach. In actuality, the difference between the two approaches is often arbitrary and is superficially imposed, hence creating the dichotomy. The two are as interrelated and interdependent as knowledge and understanding; as deduction and induction. They form an inseparable symbiotic relationship based on complimentarity. Advancements in social science are almost always the product of a joint union between idiographic understanding and nomothetic knowledge. An example of this synthesis is found in the Rorschach method: the nomothetic and idiographic approaches are merged through the use of an inductive empirical paradigm which employs objective quantifiable variables in combination with the subjective and projective responses of individuals.

Theoretical constructs are incomplete unless they can be directly related to personal lives. Knowledge, like theory, is impotent when divorced from an individual's experiences, and only becomes vitalized when augmented by the idiographic understanding which is obtained through the case study method. Since one of the major goals of social science is to understand humankind and society, it is obvious that the socio-psychological conditions of particular individuals in particular societies must be studied. The case study is methodologically designed specifically for the analysis of the intra-psychic and social dimensions of particular people. The majority of sociological, psychological and criminological principles demand conceptualization through individualized experiences. It is by employing the paradigmatic use of the case study that this individualization is achieved. The case study represents the effort of a social scientist to observe, discover, interpret and delineate the composition and structure of the actor's world and his perception of it. By portraying the actor's category of reality via the case study, another step is taken toward the understanding of ourselves and our society.

## Appendix

The following is an outline which Dr. Lemert utilized in diagnosing his own "deviant" subjects. It is offered to the sociologist compiling the case study as a tool for gathering data. The Rosenzweig Model, which follows Lemert's, is useful as a guide in writing the case study itself.

### Lemert's Outline in Studying and Writing the Life History of a Deviant

I. The Nature of the Deviation

A. Describe in detail the ways in which the person or persons deviate from the normal. Attempt to distinguish biological variation from behavioral variation if the former is involved. Measure or informally estimate how great the deviation is.

B. Distinguish the deviation in terms of its context. Does it appear to be a symptomatic reaction, situational behavior, or is it systematic behavior?

C. If there is a subculture connected with this deviation (regardless of whether the deviant participates in it), describe the folkways, techniques and skills, and the mores. Under mores, distinguish prohibitions, permissives, and compulsives.

D. If it exists, describe the social organization associated with the deviation; describe technical groups (such as the shoplifters' organization), social and auxiliary groups; describe the various roles within the deviant organization, methods of social control used in the group, leadership, and social ranking. What is the degree of solidarity and morale of the group.

E. What is the situation in the deviant's particular environment? Does a culture and a social organization exist? What are the local variations? Primary sources within the community should be consulted, if possible, for this information.

II. The Societal Reaction to the Deviant

A. What is the general reaction to this type of deviation, acceptance, rejection, inconsistent.

B. What is the degree of social distance between deviant and community?

C. Describe the societal definitions of the deviant: attitudes, stereotypes, special folklore, and mythology centering around the deviant.

D. What is the nature of the exploitative culture? Is there exploitation by sanctioned commercial agencies, by other deviants, by illegal agencies?

E. In the public control or manipulative culture, what are the objectives of control—limited services, rehabilitation, and institutional custodial care? In evaluating the experiences of the control culture, What degree of isolation is involved; how much withdrawal stress is there? Are controls paternalistic or democratic. What are the opportunities for personal development or growth within the control jurisdiction? To what degree does experience with agencies or control over this deviation provide the individual with a role suitable for independent life in society?

III. The Natural History of the Deviant

A. Describe the childhood and adult development of the deviant. Are there any crisis points in the history at which the self-conception changed?

B. How did the family react to the deviant behavior? Was deviant behavior learned in the family?

C. Describe the special societal reaction to which the deviant was exposed. What are the regional, communal, and class variations of the reaction in the deviant's case? Has the deviant been exploited, institutionalized, or manipulated in the name of community welfare? Describe.

D. If there is a deviant social organization in the community, does the individual participate? If so, how did he begin? What is his or her status in the deviant group?

E. What sort of self-conception does the deviant have? How does this correspond with the societal definition, with the definition in the deviant group, if any?

F. Estimate the adjustment of the deviant. How much emotional conflict, anxiety, neurosis, or psychosis is there, if any? Is the deviant demoralized, parasitic, or dependent?

IV. Social Participation

A. How has the deviant's occupational status and income been affected?

B. What has the deviation done to sex and family participation?

C. Describe political, religious, educational, recreational, and other aspects of participation which have been affected by his deviation.

**Rosenzweig's Outline For Writing a Case Study**

I. Identifying Data.

Name, date of birth, age, sex, race, marital status, grade in school, occupation, names of members of family.

II. Statement of Problem.

Who is referring the case and why? What is the nature of the behavior disturbance? Who is being disturbed? Give specific examples. In some cases it may be helpful to give at this time a brief history of the evolution of the problem.

III. Congenital and Physical Factors Determining Behavior

A. *Congenital factors*

Inquire regarding insanity, feeblemindedness, epilepsy, glandular disorders, alcoholism, "nervous breakdowns," instability, etc., in the maternal and paternal relatives, parents and siblings.

B. *Physical Factors (developmental)*

Inquire regarding condition of mother during pregnancy; nature of delivery; careful history of any birth injury; childhood diseases (give course and any residual of each); accidents, convulsions, fainting spells, glandular disturbances; attitudes of parents toward health; age weaned, age of walking, talking, teething; inquire especially regarding diseases of the nervous system, encephalitis, chorea, "nervousness," nervous indigestion, prolonged sleeping spells. In addition, secure height and weight norms, and report of medical or physical examination.

IV. Environmental Forces or Situations Which Have Influenced Behavior

A. *Factors in the home*

(1) Father. Inquire regarding his own childhood experiences, his education, occupation and economic status, religion, and dominant personality traits. His attitude toward wife and siblings, i.e., kindly sympathetic, dominating democratic, hobbies, recreational interests, talents, physical characteristics, frustrations, and other important factors which may help to indicate his influence on the behavior of the client.

(2) Mother. Same as for father, and in addition inquire regarding the expression of the maternal relationship. Is it one of rejection or overprotection? Follow up, depending on the problem or the tentative hypothesis established.

(3) Siblings. Inquire regarding attitude toward each other, health, undue quarreling, rivalry, degree of closeness, schooling, present whereabouts, or occupations and activities.

(4) Physical conditions. Secure a brief chro-

chronological account of home life from birth to present time, including changes in residence, foster-home placement. Inquire regarding orderliness, cleanliness, regularity, sleeping arrangements, and facilities for recreation.

5) Method of control and supervision.

Inquire if parents openly disagree in regard to discipline. Are the parents consistent? What kind of discipline, bribes, threats, deprivations? Are they indulgent, lax, repressive, cruel, or just and sensible? Are there home duties or responsibilities?

B. *Community and cultural factors*

Inquire regarding nationality and religious background; extent of participation in church activities; political activities; economic and social status of family in community; extent to which family has accepted the dominant community culture. Inquire regarding neighborhood, if possible give delinquency or other rates, dominant nationality, economic status, types of dwellings, social controls, recreational opportunities.

C. *Educational factors*

Inquire regarding age client entered school,

record schools attended, location, grades repeated or skipped, any special difficulties in school subjects—reading, arithmetic, etc. Attitudes toward teacher, subjects liked most, extracurricular activities, evidence of leadership, rank in class, educational plans and ambitions.

D. *Occupational factors*

Inquire regarding jobs held, reasons for changing jobs, dates of change, vocational interests and ambitions. What has determined them? Inquire about special skills.

E. *Recreational factors*

Inquire regarding leisure-time activities. Are they solitary or performed with groups? Is subject sought out, tolerated, or rejected by others? Are there signs of leadership? What kinds of activities are enjoyed? Do other members of family participate? Does subject hold membership in gangs, clubs? Does subject have hobbies or special interests?

V. Reactions to Congenital, Physiological, and Environmental Forces

A. *Reactions in early childhood*

*Emotional reactions.* Inquire regarding temper tantrums and how met by parents, signs of stubbornness, suspiciousness, sulking. *Fear reactions.* Inquire as to their origin and how handled by parents, any night terrors or sleep walking. *Love reactions.* Inquire about attachment to parents, dependence, overaffection, shyness, fear, thumbsucking, nail biting, masturbation, etc.

Is subject unusually sensitive, withdrawn and secretive? Is he subject to crying or laughing spells? Does he laugh spontaneously and freely? Is he listless, distractable, hyperactive? Is he quarrelsome, impatient, selfish, cruel to other children or to animals? Is he inattentive, disinterested in surroundings, fussy, repressed, tense?

B. Reaction in later childhood and adolescence

Inquire regarding freedom of expression, dependency on parents. Is subject becoming emancipated from parental control? Is he happy in group activities? Is he predominantly happy and carefree, outgoing, extroverted? Does he have many friends, is he a leader? Is he at ease with the opposite sex, does he date? What are his dominant recreational activities? Has he had any delinquency record or any contact with law-enforcment agencies?

VI. Sources of Information

List all sources of information in order of importance (as well as amount of information received). Give name, address, and relationship to subject of each person furnishing information. Statements of persons other than the main informant should be so indicated.

List impressions of the informant. Note appearance, intelligence, personality, insight, attitudes, and cooperation. Evaluate the reliability and adequacy of the information given. Evaluate the informant's capacity, intellectually and emotionally, to cooperate in a plan of treatment of the subject.

List all social agencies who have had contact with the family (relief, medical, psychiatric, and other agencies) and the history of the contact of each. Include reports from agencies in the body of the case history under appropriate headings, indicating source in every case.

At this point, it will be helpful to examine several psychological tests which shed light on Dave's particular deviations. In their general applications, these tests illustrate how previous subjective data can be enhanced with more scientific methods.

Draw-a-Person Test

A Draw-a-Person Test (similar to the Rorschach Ink Blot and the Thematic Apperception Test) is a graphic means of portraying personality through an individual's projections. Self-expressions reveal inner conflicts, self-conceptions, psychic values, psycho-sexual and psycho-social tensions. "The basic assumption verified repeatedly in clinical experience is that the human figure drawn by an individual who is instructed to 'draw a person' relates intimately to the impulses, anxieties, conflicts, and compensations characteristic of that individual. In some sense, the figure *is* the individual." (Mackover 1949, 37.) The picture drawn can be viewed as a symbolic representation of the artist's psyche. Therefore, every detail in the drawing is significant: theme, action, movement, succession, symmetry, perspective, stance, position, anatomical structures, facial features, type of lines, and size and placement. The following drawings and statments concerning the drawings by the subject are exceedingly representational and demonstrative. They lucidly reveal his bisexuality, diffuse identity, anxiety and hostility. When asked to comment on his first drawing, he stated that the person in the drawing was "... a son of the Gods ... of both sexes, mostly a male ... someone who is fighting, striving and always looking up." The Icarus theme is evident here in the upward direction and movement of the bodies against the sun, in the striving action, and in his statment about the form being "... a son of the Gods...." The first two pictures display a person moving and striving upward, yet being restrained from advancing freely. Beyond this disorganized, self-defeating striving, the subject's diffuse identity is accentuated by the reinforced lines delineating the person's bodily boundaries. The contours of the body lines are overly-stressed and overly-determined.

This over-emphasis on bodily boundaries could be explained in terms of early psychosexual development. In the early stages (especially in the oral stage) the subject attempted to delineate and differentiate between himself and his environment (between his mother's breast and his ego boundary). Due to the domineering personality of the subject's mother, this process of separating self from external objects was impaired. Consequently, the subject developed poorly cathected ego-boundaries and a weak sense of self, which is represented in all of the following drawings.

Leading the hierarchy of anatomical parts, the head in each picture was drawn first. Thus, the head contains the central location of the subject's "self." His drawings are all overly head-oriented, emphasizing the head so markedly in fact, that in drawing #3 he tore through the page. The drawing of the heads was always done forcefully and aggressively. This emphasis reflects the subject's drug usage, for the purpose of ingesting a drug may be to obfuscate and narcotize the "head." The drug argot refers to users as "heads"—"pot heads," "acid heads" and the like—and the subject frequently uses terms such as "playing head games," "getting my head straight," and "head talk." The effects of drugs prevent thinking—"like having a marshmellow inside my head" or "a balloon inside my skull." In all but the first drawings, the faces were left featureless and, even in the first, the features are so vague as to be almost undiscernable (i.e., eyes and mouth represented by two lines).

According to Mackover (1949, 40):

> The subject who deliberately omits facial features in a drawing showing careful and often aggressive delineation of contour and detail of other parts of the figure is one who is often evasive about the frictional character of his interpersonal relationships. This treatment is a graphic expression of an avoidance of the problem. Superficially, caution and hostility may characterize the social contacts of the individual.

It is most significant that the facial features are missing because of the extreme social importance centered about the head. The head is the only bodily part which is always exposed and is the initiator and recipient of social actions. What the subject chooses to put on the blank page represents his thematic apperception of his environment: in each drawing, self-absorption and autocentricity dominate the central theme. The subject used the entire page for drawing the persons and left very little space blank.

Another central theme is the overly-determined, aggressively drawn boundaries of each figure's contour. Each person's body outline was heavily drawn and redrawn as if a strict defintion would separate the person from his environment.

## I. Drawing #1, time—3:25 minutes

Subject was instructed to "Draw a person and then tell me about that person."

Statements concerning the figure: (1) "It's a son of the Gods." (2) "It's both sexes, mostly a male." (3) "It's striving, fighting and always looking up." (4) "It's radiating all this energy." (5) "Everything is very powerful—feelings, energy, life, and death."

**II. Drawing #2, time—2:57 minutes**

Subject was instructed to "Now draw a person of the opposite sex and then tell me about that person."

Statements concerning the figure: (1) "It's a female." (2) "It's kind of tied-up—bound or chained to something." (3) "... digs sex a lot, but likes it hard and forceful." (4) "It's very intense, extremely intense!" (5) "... bubbling, juicy, passionate...." (6) "It's about to explode sexually."

**III. Drawing #3, time—2:00 minutes**

Subject was instructed to "Draw a person with your eyes closed."

No statements concerning figure.

**IV. Drawing #4, time—3:00 minutes**

Subject was instructed to "Draw a person who is lying down."

No statments concerning figure.

Cue-(Q) Sort Test

The purpose of this Q-sort test is to validate my observation and conclusions concerning the subject's personality characteristics. A Q-sort test is composed of one hundred cards containing a myriad of statements concerning personality and behavioral characteristics (e.g., "Is a genuinely dependable and responsible person," or "Is productive; gets things done," and so on). A judge will sort the cards, categorizing them into nine positions, ranging from "most characteristic" to "least characteristic." The subject in this case was judged by three people: (A) myself, (B) an acquaintance of the subject who had previously read the case history, and (C) a reader of the case history. In order for a Q-sort to be valid, there must be a minimum correlation between the judges of .30. The following are the three resultant correlations among the three judges: Judge A—Judge B: .35; Judge A—Judge C: .57; Judge B—Judge C: .62.

The following are the statements found "most characteristic" for Dave:

1. Is self-defeating.

2. Tends to perceive many different contexts in sexual terms; eroticizes situations.

3. Is subtly negativistic; tends to undermine and obstruct or sabotage.

4. Feels cheated and victimized by life; self-pitying.

5. Tends to project his own feelings and motivations onto others.

6. Concerned with own adequacy as a person, either at conscious or unconscious levels.

7. Feels lack of personal meaning in life.

8. Has hostility toward others.

9. Interprets basically simple and clear-cut situations in complicated and particularized ways.

10. Seeks reassurance from others.

11. Has high aspiration level for self.

12. Is basically distrustful of people in general, questions their motivations.

13. Tends to be rebellious and non-conforming.

14. Enjoys sensuous experiences (including touch, taste, smell, physical contact).

15. Is introspective and concerned with self as an object.

16. Tends to ruminate and have persistent, preoccupying thoughts.

17. Does not vary roles, relates to everyone in the same way.

18. Has insight into own motives and behavior.

19. Appears to have a high degree of intellectual capacity.

20. Reluctant to commit self to any definite course of action; tends to delay or avoid action.

21. Is concerned with own body and the adequacy of its physiological functioning.

22. Appears straightforward, forthright, candid in dealing with others.

23. Is physically attractive; good-looking.

The following are the statements found "least characteristic":

1. Is a genuinely dependable and responsible person.

2. Behaves in a giving way toward others.

3. Has a wide range of interests.

4. Tends to be self-defensive.

5. Is skilled in social techniques of imaginative play, pretending and humor.

6. Behaves in a sympathetic or considerate manner.

7. Tends to over-control needs and impulses, binds tensions excessively; delays gratification unnecessarily.

8. Is productive; gets things done.

9. Is turned to for advice and reassurance.

10. Is facially and/or gesturally expressive.

11. Emphasizes being with others; gregarious.

12. Behaves in an ethically consistent manner; is consistent with own personal standards.

13. Is subjectively unaware of self-concern; feels satisfied with self.

14. Has a clear-cut, internally consistent personality.

15. Appears straightforward, forthright, candid in dealing with others.

16. Is cheerful.

17. Handles anxiety and conflicts by refusing to recognize their presence; repressive or dissociative tendencies.

18. Is personally charming.

19. Is self-dramatizing; histrionic.

20. Favors conservative values in a variety of areas.

21. Is protective to those close to him.

22. Is genuinely submissive; accepts domination comfortably.

23. Has a rapid personal tempo; behaves and acts quickly.

The Minnesota Multiphasic Personality Inventory

The MMPI is used to obtain scores on the most important traits of personality. It is a psychometric measure. Traits that are commonly characterized as disabling are tabulated. The test itself consists of 550 statements covering subject matter from physical environment to social attitudes (Hathaway 1942, 5).

The following areas render the subject's higher scores: (1) Deviance, marked by rebelliousness against authority. (2) Low self-esteem, marked by self-deprecation and lack of self-confidence. (3) Negative self-concept, marked by a history of destructive experiences.

The Sentence Completion Test

According to Rotter (1947, 305) who created the Sentence Completion Test, the test can reveal an individual's "feelings towards his family and past drives, his inner states, goals, cathexes, reactions to frustration and failure, time perception, optimism or pessimism, and his reactions toward others."

The subject was urged "to complete the sentences as quickly as possible with the first thought that comes to mind that expresses personal feelings." Except for numbers 24 and 37, he proceeded rapidly and steadily. It is very significant that conflict and blocking occurred here; number 24 ("The future....") presented the unknown and the unstructured while number 37 ("I....") required a decision concerning his feelings about himself. Rotter (op. cit., 307) believes that "erasures and omissions frequently appear where individuals feel that their responses have been too revealing or when an item has touched upon a critical area."

Other critical and conflicted areas were revealed: (1) Negative self-concept. The subject's statements reveal his negativistic attitudes toward himself: #9, "What annoys me–is myself," #5, "I regret–my actions," #27, "I am best when–I'm high," and #29, "What pains me–is myself." In general, his statements stress negatives rather than positives, reflecting his fatalistic orientation. (2) Fatalism. Dave blocked on answering #24, "The future is...," perhaps because it looked so bleak to him. His references to the possibilities of change were doubtful: #39, "My greatest worry–is I can't change," and #15, "I can't–give up." The underlying current thought in most of the sentences is that of dysphoric mood. The success-failure syndrome of Icarus is evidenced by #36, "I secretly—want to be great," and #33, "The only trouble—myself." (3) Aggressiveness. As he did in the Draw-a-Person Test, the subject here again pressed very heavily upon the paper. He felt the need to exert strong pressure upon his environment. However, although he displayed outward manifestations of aggressiveness, he is latently passive-dependent. He states while discussing his wife, "I don't know what I'd do if I didn't have her to fall back on." (4) Psychic energy displaced. The subject de-emphasizes his past, #2, "The happiest time—is yet to come," #8, "The best—is yet to come," and #11, "A mother—was bad"), ignores the present, and describes an ambiguous future. The subject expends too much psychic energy either recreating past unresolved conflicts or fantasizing about the future. The present is too threatening and unsatisfying for interaction, consequently, the past or future are perceived as safer areas with which to cope.

The following are Dave's responses (in italics) to the Sentence Completion Test:

1. I like *art.*

2. The happiest time *is yet to come.*

3. I want to know *more about myself.*

4. Back home *was bad.*

5. I regret *my actions.*

6. At bedtime *I masturbate.*

7. Boys *are nice.*
8. The best *is yet to come.*
9. What annoys me *is myself.*
10. People *can be shits.*
11. A mother *was bad.*
12. I feel *okay.*
13. My greatest fear *is fear itself.*
14. In high school *I succeeded.*
15. I can't *give up.*
16. Sports *are fun.*
17. When I was a child *I was hung up.*
18. My nerves *are shot.*
19. Other people *bother me.*
20. I suffer *a lot.*
21. I failed *a lot.*
22. Reading *interests me.*
23. My mind *is complicated.*
24. The future *?*
25. I need *strength.*
26. Marriage *is frightening.*
27. I am best when *I'm high.*
28. Sometimes *I want to give up.*
29. What pains me *is myself.*
30. I hate *stupid people.*
31. This school *is groovey.*

32. I am very *intelligent.*
33. The only trouble *is myself.*
34. I wish *I could change.*
35. My father *was a whimp* [sic].
36. I secretly *want to be great.*
37. I *?*
38. Dancing *is boring.*
39. My greatest worry is *I can't change.*
40. Most girls *are sexy.*

Word-Association Test

It is evident in this Word-Association Test, in the subject's lack of spontaneity in answering and in his constant use of words like "death," "kill," "blood," "rape," and so on, that he is attempting to fulfill his definition of himself as a disturbed, "sick" person.

The following are Dave's responses (following hyphen) to the Word-Association Test:

world-globe

love-hate

father-son

hat-hard

breast-blood

curtains-death

trunk-vagina

drink-cold

party-pooper
bowel movement-fornication
book-bleed
lamp-shade
rug-death
chair-bleed
boy friend-girl friend
penis-hurt
dark-scarey [sic]
depressed-depressed
spring-summer
bowl-sing
suicide-the end
mountain-the end
house-womb
paper-sale
homosexual-me
radiator-warmth
girl friend-boy friend
screen-screen
masturbate-death
frame-reference
man-love
orgasm-death
movies-pretty

cut-cunt
laugh-die
bite-bleed
woman-killer
dance-sing
dog-cat
daughter-sorrow
taxi-yellow
mother-fucker
table-top
beef-jerky
nipple-breast
race-eternity
water-fountain
suck-sick
horse-powerful
fire-powerful
vagina-blood
farm-alone
social-want
son-warmth
taxes-stupid
tobacco-stimulating
city-impersonal
intercourse-impersonal

hospital-bed
doctor-death

Historical Data on Dave

I. Family History:

A. Parents. Caucasian, high school graduates, borderline lower-middle class. Social values are lower class. Father is a sheet metal laborer, mother does general office work, works in a bakery, and is a part-time call girl.

Mother

Interests: sex, clothes

Temperament: open-minded, boisterous

Health: normal

Characteristics: over-solicitous, anxious, possessive, domineering

Father

Interests: gardening

Temperament: narrow-minded, quiet

Health: heart attacks

Characteristics: indifferent, passive, negativistic

In general, the home atmosphere was never really harmonious. Prior to the divorce, there was a great deal of discourse; only afterwards was there semi-harmony. The home was essentially matriarchal. Dave's younger brother (and only sibling) was indifferent, resembling the father in his attitudes. Dave was given free choice as to religious instruction—he is an atheist of Jewish and Russian Orthodox background. His special enjoyments at home, as he recalls, were masturbation when alone, or working with clay models. There was a large and non-harmonious family circle: Dave disliked his grandparents and other relations intensely. Dave's family lived in a poor section of east Los Angeles prior to moving to a lower-middle class neighborhood in west Los Angeles where he began junior high school.

B. Brother. Dave has one brother three years younger, whom he described as quiet and hostile (taking after his father in that he has resented Dave for his entire life). Dave feels superior to his brother.

II. Personal History: Born 3/23/43, a natural birth. Does not recall time of weaning. First remembered experience: sexual play with neighborhood girls at age two or three. Dave does not recall parents during early years.

III. Illnesses and Habits: Pneumonia and general weak health, nightmares, finicky with food.

IV. School and College: Entered kindergarten at age five, graduated college at 22. Dave was best at science and math, poor in English. Dave had few friendships; he was shy, submissive, and introverted. Dave had hero-worship for a science teacher in junior high school, because of the teachers intelligence.

V. Sex History: Early curiosity, first learned of sexual relations between parents at age fifteen—remembers being "shocked." During youth, Dave practiced masturbation, but did not engage in self-display. He "liked looking at young girls' vaginas." During puberty, Dave fell in love, first with a boy, then with a girl—"with people similar to myself." Dave's erotic fantasies consisted of the destruction of a woman and controlling and inflicting pain on her. Dave also fantasized himself as being raped. His ideal mate he described as "a beautiful woman with same goals as myself and with money." His emotions following sexual experiences were often guilt and worries of potency. Dave's attitudes toward marriage consisted of the desire for a new type of marriage with new rules—rules in relation to mutual need and not society's—that would allow extramarital dating, of both sexes.

VI. Major Experiences: On the positive side, Dave's childhood memory was "When I got a set of toy six guns for Hanukah." During adolescence, "when my science teacher [father surrogate] took me to Mexico for a summer and took me away from my home and showed me a different life. He also helped me through school, teaching interesting things in the physical sciences, but my mother sensed he was queer, and broke the ties between us. He changed me from being a hood." During young adulthood, Dave's positive memory was going to Europe. In this, he felt that he had achieved something he never thought he could attain. "I was really jealous of you [meaning me] when you went and I hated you for it."

On the negative side, during childhood, Dave cites strained relations between his parents, "The whole situation with my father and mother before they got separated was depressing—one continual fight." During adolescence, Dave cited the "loss of a close friend, who forsook me for his girl." During young adulthood, Dave felt like an outsider, "Not being able to get along with my peer group in high school; felt rejection of my advances by the girls. I was in an outgroup because I was poor."

VII. Aims and Aspirations: Dave says that he'd like "to be great—in any sense—to be a God ... I'd like to be the Messiah—the bringer of happiness to everyone and to myself." Dave wishes for "love, greatness, money." Dave's estimate of self and world that the world is "rejecting because of its own fears of my inherent badness ... I want love from everyone and have to reject old lovers for new ones." For Dave the world's attitude toward him is "fearful and upset by my outgoing attitudes." He estimates himself as intelligent, over and beyond most people. Dave feels his special qualities make him a special person, "I'm extremely sensitive and have a tremendous need for love ... I am closer to being crazy than most people because I'm more aware of what's happening inside my head ... because I don't repress ... and I'm artistic."

## Sociological and Criminological Interpretations of Non-Directive Interview

Taped interviews (non-directive and directive) were conducted over a period of three weeks. The following excerpts are my summaries of Dave's spontaneous (undirected) comments and reflections. The excerpts do not read as a continuous story, largely because Dave's reflections were not chronologically or substantively organized.

Tape #1:

counter 005:

Born and lives in East Los Angeles, a slum characterized by minority groups, disorganization, and high crime rates.

033:

Moves to West Los Angeles and enters a middle-class school where he comes into contact with middle-class values and wealth symbols.

040:

Parent's affection toward him is lacking: His mother is neurotic and destructive, his father is absent and has a lack concern for children.

043:

Parents separated and subject lives with mother.

047:

Parents constantly fighting.

050:

Malicious, non-utilitarian behavior "... going out for kicks—stealing and wrecking"—which is not done out of need.

079:

"We'd even cheat among ourselves when playing cards."

206:

"She'd [Dave's mother] steal groceries, etc. Her friends turned me on to pot. My father would make me watch for cops when he'd steal gas."

232:

Takes drugs for definite reasons—to sleep or to relieve tension and acute nervousness. But masochistic, hedonistic drug use is stressed, "to punish myself 'cuz the come-down on that stuff is terrible."

333:

Eventually Dave's basic trust is shattered, "That's when I first realized you can't believe in anyone; my best friend turned me in."

425:

Dave discovered the effects of demerol in a hospital. This supports the theory (Felix 1954) that accidental and medical types of addicts become addicted through extended drug use in a hospital. Dave's experience also supports Isbell's notion of psychoneurotic types who seek to relieve their anxieties and psychopaths who seek release of their unconscious aggressive drives and hostility against society.

436:

Lindesmith's theory (1940) of opiatic addiction (that addiction occurs when the user is able to identify and define withdrawal symptoms with the drug), is supported by Dave's own admission, "I'd beg and scream, call the nurse for another shot—I wanted a shot like I never wanted a shot before in my life. My head was 'straight'—nobody bothered me—but the come-down, wow!"

450:

Merton's (1964) theory of retreatist-double-failure, where the drug use is an escape from the failure in both the legitimate and illegitimate world, is illustrated in Dave's case, "I learned it was a good escape."

774:

"It makes things a lot nicer; reality sometimes can be fake-reality [with drugs]... reality can be too real; it's seeing it without the emotion. When things get too bad, it acts as a buffer."

848:

Takes drug to fight neurotic anxieties, "I flipped out cold, seeing things coming out of the walls—really paranoid—extremely paranoid and frightened; scared out of my mind for three days!!"

878:

Early sexual experiences such as rape fantasies, violence, and homosexual experiences.

**Interpretations of Directive Interview**

The following excerpts are from directive interviews in which I pressed Dave to follow up on incomplete or fragmentary thoughts, especially as these pertained to the concerns in Lemert's outline and in Rosenzweig's outline.

Tape #2

038:

Feels guilty after anal intercourse with homosexual partner and breaks up the relationship with him.

050:

Wakes up at night with global fear (while in Europe); feels the fear was related to homosexual experience, and then relates it to the same fear he felt as a child–such as fear of monsters. Castration anxiety.

064:

Experiences identity crisis whic reveals subject's high degree of suggestibility: laughs and can't look at me, "Monsters, grotesque and unidentifiable ... I couldn't identify myself."

093:

Father was away in the war and Dave lived with his mother for the first five or six years of his life, never having seen his father. Dave speaks of a strange monster coming back and taking love of mother away from subject, which he had possessed exclusively.

111:

Mother recently displays seductive tendencies toward Dave, "Feel my breasts and look at my vagina to see if I have cancer."

130:

Subject's interpretation of sex is heavily laden with switches of sexual identity and death, "I like to inflict pain in my fantasies about women." When engaged in homosexual activities, Dave fantasizes being the woman, "... ramming a giant phallus into a womb, or rape scenes, bloody."

160:

Mother is inconsistent in giving love.

194:

Mother is omnipresent figure in thoughts about other women, "I couldn't marry the girl I loved because I'm too dependent and untrusting and afraid ... worrying she wouldn't be there ...." This refers perhaps to mothers desertion at father's return.

216:

Sex is continually identified with violence, "Orgasms, the more they hurt, the more I like them."

226:

The subject identifies with his mother, "I am the girl being screwed in my fantasy."

260:

Dreams of making love with a huge frightening monster, getting enveloped and attacked. Takes drugs to sooth these terrifying thoughts, and which allow him to sleep.

290:

Mother would fix up the subject and his friends with prostitutes and would coerce the subject into bringing boy friends, girlfriends, and club meetings to their house, making sure that she was included. She would say degrading things about girls, knowing that he would not fall in love with a prostitute. This way, she would keep his love.

337:

Trying to identify with his father: the latter is passive, but he supposedly "raped" his mother on their wedding night, and she bled. The subject in his rape fantasies of women is trying to identify with the only "masculine" thing his father ever did.

340:

Regression to the first narcissistic stage: transforming his sex partner (while under the influence of drugs) into himself, making love to himself. The subject has trouble loving because of this regressive tendency, which prevents him from forming object relationships.

367:

Mother makes him feel guilty about being male.

378:

Mother was against Dave's marriage and tried to stop it.

412:

On taking marijuana: "When its even for kicks, I know I really do it out of frustration."

435:

On sexual ambivalence: "One long chain of words comes to my mind when having orgasms ... fly, gold, wild, goose, egg, dog, cat, fight, die, kill, power, gold, go sing, sorrow, happy, yes, no, I don't know, happy-o, sad-o, come, go."

481:

Subject painted picture of a man going into the sun (representing the womb), "Bright yellow light, gold and beautiful, and I was part of it," and of giant hands (superego, society) which held him back.

482:

Dave reveals suicidal tendencies; he mentions his feelings of having no control over his body as he walks toward the San Francisco Bay (water, womb, mother).

490:

At this point the subject smokes three marijuana cigarettes.

500:

Erotic stimulation from body.

529:

"I'm there, in the big cavity."

588:

Death/rebirth scene—the subject wants to reborn.

650:

Figures created by the subject in his paintings and sculptures symbolize his desire to return to the womb. He creates these without preplanning or forethought, "I just feel an urge to paint or sculpt and I go ahead and try to figure them out later." On a recent painting, "A man is reaching with one outstretched arm for a return to the womb (or death, away from the world) and the other is holding on to the hands of society (or his father, his super-ego) which is asking him to stop."

691:

"Once I'm in something, I have to pretend it's the best thing I'm in, cuz it's the only thing I'm in, and if I say anything about it, I'll feel terribly guilty, and won't be honest with the thing I'm in or the person."

722:

"The world's too harsh."

740:

"The fucking thing is enveloping me, and I'm in it now! All these lights, oh, God, I don't know what I'm going to do; I don't know how to get out, I'm a globe, and I'm getting smaller!"

[The following pages were typed by the subject while under the influence of demerol–sic.]

Now things are vecoming very aware to me. I see that i'm not doing all i can to idolate myself form other people. all other people. I think its because i dont want to love anyone or that i really cant , that i dont know how to cope with love so i'm trying be bext to keep away form it. I really enjoy this feeling of lonliness i want it i dont want an yone at ll , all i want is myself. i thik. or i do want some one, but dont know haw to give love back once its given tome. i'm rejecting all of the relationships i have with anyone now. even judy, i'm talking myself into believeing that sehe really does not love me at all, but really hates me because i'm such a shit. this is probably my feelings i have with my mother, ive. i've only learned to cope with a rejection from her, a lack of love, so i martyr myself as to only get love thru sympathy, which my mother does. I'm making myself very alone so as to get that same feeling over agin that i used to have. that feeling of pleasure in knowing that i can , realy have the power to repulse people. when i'm in situation where my repulsive acts dont work, i get shook up and dont like the situation because i no longer have the power to destroy the love of others, that's all i really get pleasure out of doing, destroying a love htat others have given me. Being in that position where i can make the other person feel guilty for not being able to give me some ,enough love. So indirectly i destroy them at the same time as i make them feel as though they did it to me. Where in actuality i'm the one who really destroyed the relationship, soon as I say that i had the upper hand in the situation. Or as soon as i saw myself getting to close to being able to reci procate the love. If i can only find out why i do this then maybe i can fight it and then be able to have a real meaningful relationship with outhers. I am doing this with dan, i told him he was the one that caused our first break in high school, where in actuality it was probably my doing it to him. Because he had the audacity ot love me, me a real shit, full of hate for the world and the peole in it. Me the one who can only manipulate others for my own means, and when i cant do htat, i get out or hert the other person real bad because they refute my power , that all dominating force in my life, to be greater than anyone else in the world. to be *THE DESTROYER. not the creator.* to be the killer not the giver not the lover not the wise helpful one, but the iffinite bad one the hate one. Mybe all this that i'm saying is all bull shit in that i'm just feeling taribly guilty for some thing that ive done. Maybe that some thing is the constant lying i do with people in telling them i love them and really knowing inside that i really dont. and that i really have only selfishe fellings of just wanting to get their love on a one way basis. I think this may be the case, because i notice my feelings of guilt in almost every situation where a new person comes into view that i have feelings for. I see myself liking them and then i notice that i no longer care AT ALL about the first person i was with and now focus all of my attention on the new person. and so feel guilty and hateful towards the original person.

I alsays fin d myself in this posituion with oeople, jum, dan, judy, steve, suzin, etc. But i cant do anything aboutit , i just continue knowing that im doing it, and then after feel very guilty. I hope that i really want to know why i do this things. But i sort of feel that i really want to know, i want to continue on being this self destructive way, maybe its because i feeli my life has been so bad that i want to kill myself, and that yhis is a very subtle way of doing it, ie. forcing myself into such strong feelings of guilt that i will then, driven by intense passion against myself kill myself and get my ultimate wish of "happiness" and Peace.

But why do i want to kill myself so bad? Why do i keep forcing myself into such an awful position. Maybe if i find out whi i will then be able to change my life to live it instead of die it. Because is notice that everything that i do now is orienter toward the suidical act. I'm now smoking an awfilly lot, knowing that it may give me cancer and enevitable death, and yet still i continue onn, like subly hoping th t it will. I also want o get amotorcycle which iv very death oriented. I also stopped eating for a long time knowing th t it would destroy my health and possible enevityably death. I also have this urinal infection which i wont go to a doctor about, i keep making rationalizations about it and putting it off—so as tb perpetuated the malignancy. and when i'm riding my vycycle i keep thinking of what it would be like to get run over, flying through the air into my last peace—the end. But why why why do i do this , i know what i'm doing, but i cant seem to stop myself, i just carry on with the steps toward death. WHY?........

Ive just talked myself away from my feelings of love, very ingeniusly. or i'm now talking myself away from my suicidal feeling. any way i want to get back to me need for love. I seem to have this unfillable need for love, i'm hapiest when i'm getting it from everyone, and not hurting anyones feelings. but soon as it stops i feel that i' m lost again, or guilty again, and therfore the suicidal tendancyies. I guess maybe that is it, i feel guilty about wanting to get love from all people all of the time. And soon as i stop getting it in the slightest way i dont really get mad at the other person, but turn it in and get mad at myself. I guess i really do get mad at the others when they stop giving me love- in fact i hate them and want to kill them for it those sone of a bitches. those fucking bastards—i hate them all alll alll—non ofe than are no damn good (for love that is).

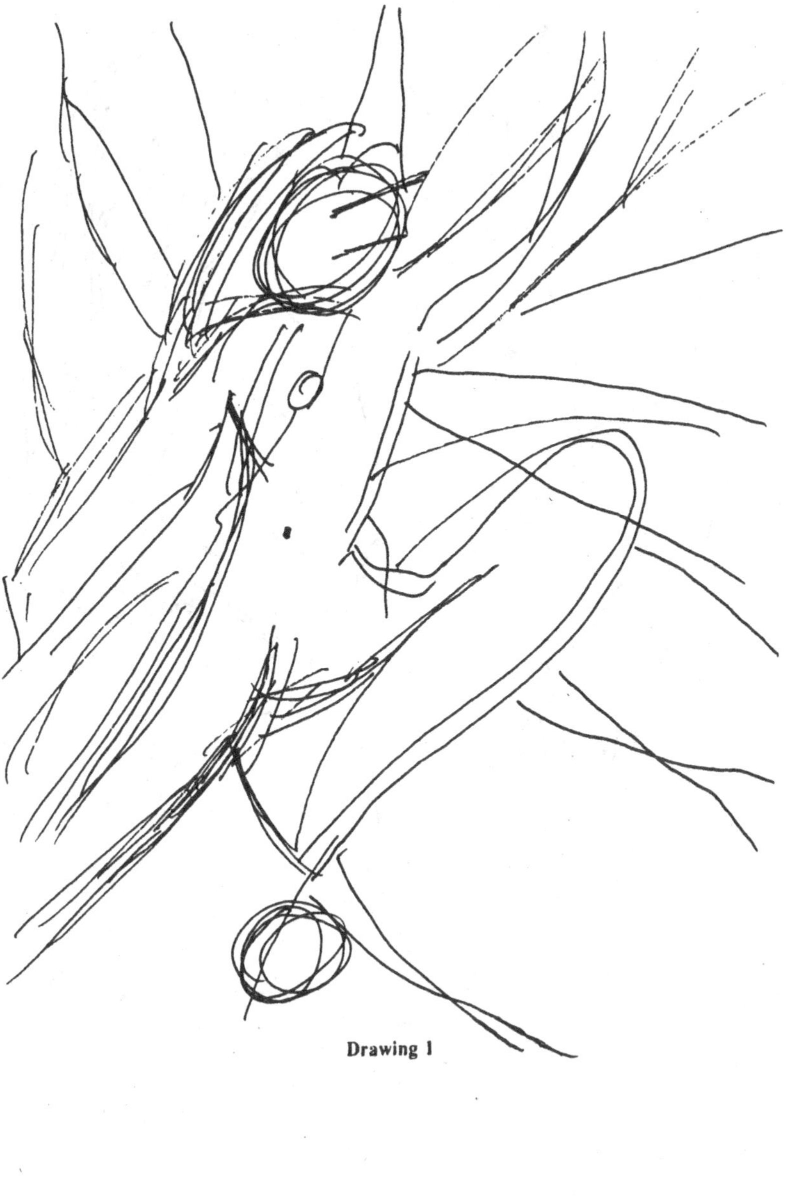

Drawing 1

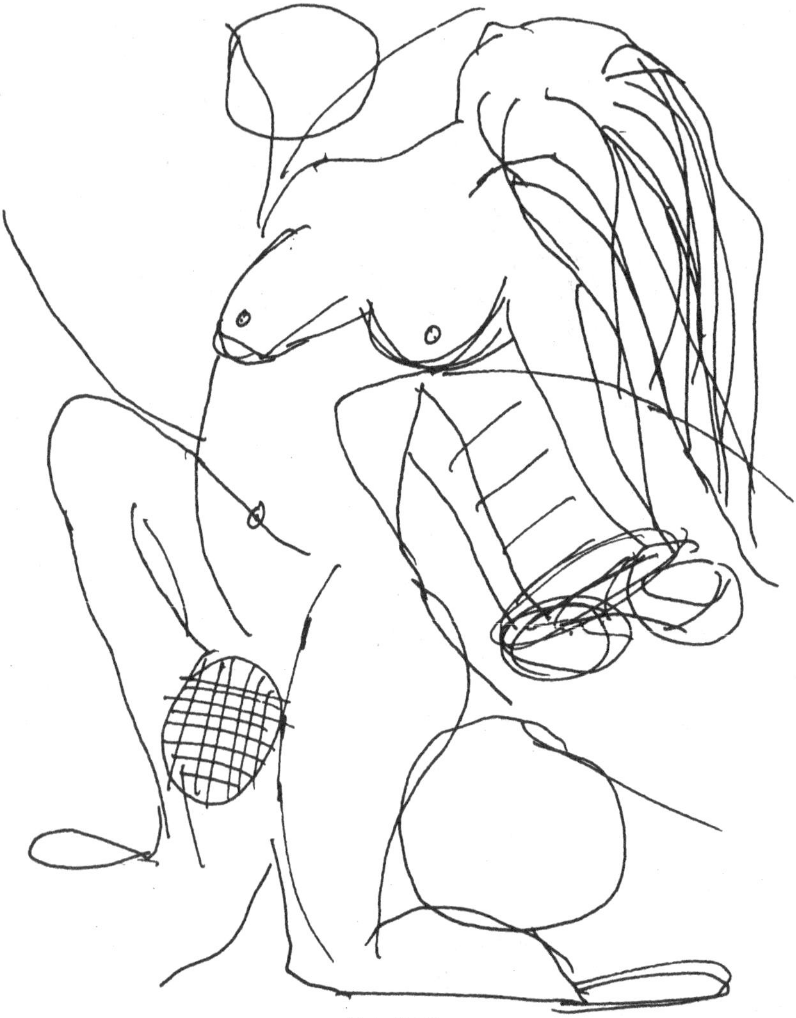

**Drawing 2**

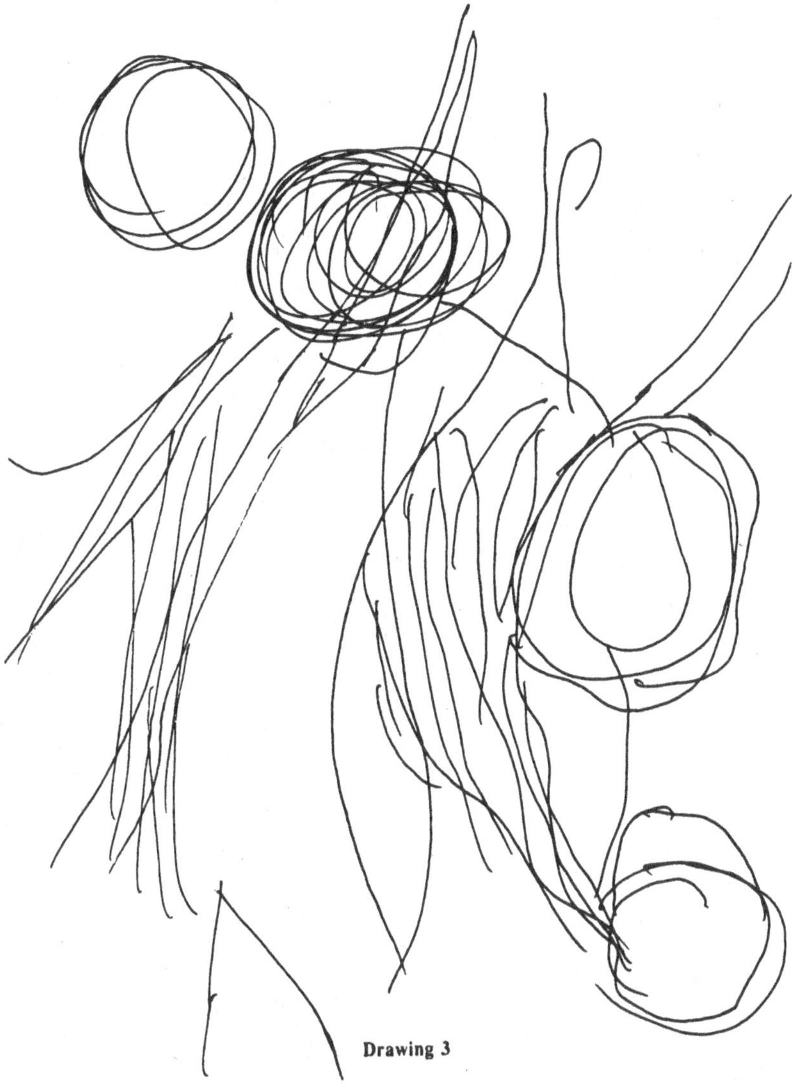

**Drawing 3**

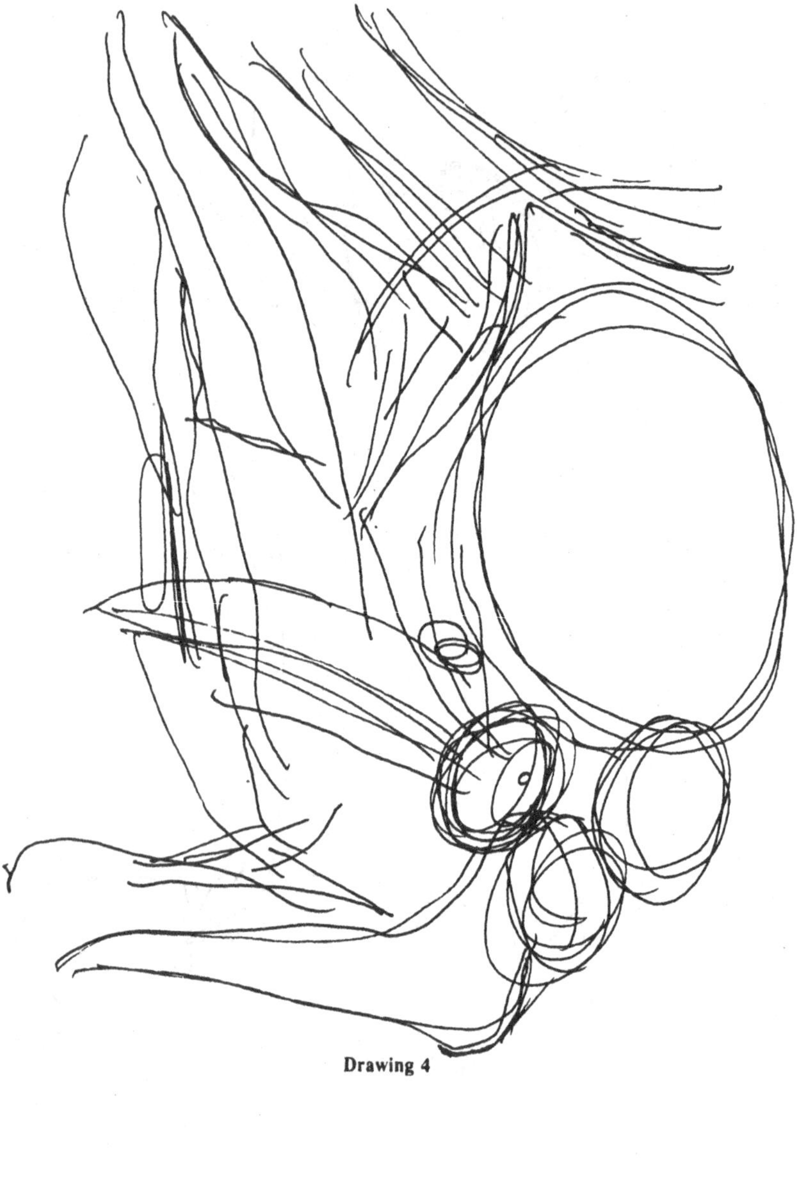

Drawing 4

## Bibliography


Abel, T. "The Nature and Use of Biograms." *American Journal of Sociology*, 53 (1947), 111-118.

Abercrombie, M. L. J. *The Anatomy of Judgement*. New York: Basic Books, 1960.

Adler, A. *The Case of Miss R.* New York: Greenburg, 1929.

Alexander, F. "A Study of the Psychotherapeutic Process." Paper read at the Western Division Meeting of the American Psychiatric Association, Los Angeles. Nov. 1957.

Allport, G. W. "The Use of Personal Documents in Psychological Science." *Social Science Research Council Bulletin*, 49 (1942).

______. *Becoming*. New Haven: Yale University Press, 1955.

______. *Pattern and Growth in Personality*. New York: Holt, 1961.

______, J. S. Bruner, and E. M. Jandorf. "Personality Under Social Catastrophe: An Analysis of 90 German Refugee Life Histories." *Character and Personality*, 10 (1941), 1-22.

______, and E. P. Vernon. *Studies in Expressive Movement*. New York: Macmillan, 1933.

Anderson and Anderson. *An Introduction to Projective Techniques*. New York: Prentice-Hall, 1951.

Angell, R. C. and R. Freeman. "The Use of Documents, Records, Census Materials, and Indices." In

*Research Methods in the Behavioral Sciences.* Ed. L. Festinger and D. Katz. New York: Dryden Press, 1953.

Angyal, A. *Neurosis and Treatment: A Holistic Theory.* New York: John Wiley and Sons, 1965.

Anonymous. *A Young Girl's Diary.* Prefaced by Sigmund Freud. New York: Thomas Seitzer, 1921.

Armitage, G. H. "Barbituate Addiction and Sensitivity." *British Journal of Medicine,* 33 (December, 1960), 149-155.

Asch, P. "The Reliability of Psychiatric Diagnosis." *Journal of Abnormal Psychology,* 44 (1949), 272-276.

Ausubel, D. P. *Drug Addiction: Physiological, Psychological and Sociological Aspects.* New York: Glencoe Free Press, 1958.

Baldwin, A. L. "The Statistical Analysis of the Structure of a Single Personality." *Psychological Bulletin,* 37 (1940).

Bateson, G. and D. Jackson. "The Genesis of Mental Disorders and Social Deviance." *Behavioral Science,* 1 (1956), 251-264.

Bechterew, W. *New Studies in Reflexology and Physiology of the Nervous System.* 1925.

Beck, S. J. "Rorschach's Erlebnistypus: An Empiric Datum." *Separata aus Beheft zur Schweiz., Z. Psychol. Rorschachiana,* 7:45, 1963.

Becker, E. *The Revolution in Psychiatry.* New York: Glencoe Free Press, 1964.

______. *The Birth and Death of Meaning.* New York: Glencoe Free Press, 1962.

Becker, H. *Outsiders.* New York: Glencoe Free Press, 1963.

______, and A. Strauss. "Careers, Personality, and Adult Socialization." *American Journal of Sociology,* 62 (November, 1956), 254-263.

Beers, C. W. *A Mind that found Itself: An Autobiography.* New York: Doran, 1938.

Bell, D. "The Rediscovery of Alienation: Some Notes Along the Quest for the Historical Marx." *Journal of Philosophy,* 56 (November, 1959).

Bell, W. "Anomie, Social Isolation, and the Class Structure." *Sociometry,* 20 (June, 1957), 105-116.

Berg, C. and C. Allen. *The Problem of Homosexuality: Disease of a Way of Life.* New York: Hill and Wong, 1957.

Berger, Peter. *Invitation to Sociology: A Humanistic Perspective.* New York: Doubleday, 1963.

Bettelheim, B. *My Life in Nazi Concentration Camps.* Girard, Kansas: Julius Haldeman, 1960.

Biber, I. et al. *Homosexuality.* New York: Basic Books, 1962.

Bingham, W. V. and B. V. Moore. *How to Interview.* New York: Harper, 1941.

Bleicher, Josef. *The Hermeneutic Imagination: Outline of a Positive Critique of Scientism and Sociology.* London: RKP, 1982.

Block, J. "A Comparison Between Ipsative and Normative Ratings of Personality." *Journal of Abnormal Sociology,* 54 (1957), 50-54.

Blumer, Herbert. "Critiques of Research in the Social Sciences: An Appraisal of Thomas and Znaniecki's *The Polish Peasant." Social Science Research Council, Bulletin*, 44 (1939).

Bolgar, H. "The Case Study Method." *Handbook of Clinical Psychology*. Ed. B. Wolman. New York: Hill Book Co., 1965.

Bolgar, Hedda. "The Structure of Emotional Experience in the Course of Human Life." Ph.D. Dissertation. Vienna, 1934.

Bonaparte, M. "A Defense of Biography." *International Journal of Psycho-Analysis*, 20 (1939), 231-240.

Breuer, J. and Sigmund Freud. *Studies in Hysteria*. New York: Basic Books, 1957.

Bryman, Alan. "The Debate About Quantitative Research: A Question of Method or Epistemology." *British Journal of Sociology*, 35:1 (1984), 75-92.

Bugental, J. F. T. and S. L. Zelen. "Investigations into the Self-Concept." *Journal of Personality*, 18 (1950), 483-498.

Burgess, E. W. "What Social Case Records Should Contain To Be Useful for Logical Interpretation." *Social Forces*, 6 (June, 1928), 524-532.

Burney, C. *Solitary Confinement*. New York: Coward-McCann, 1952.

Butler, J. M., N. Laura, and Alice K. Wagstaff. "On the Naturalistic Definition of Variables: An Analogue of Clinical Analysis." *Research in Psycho-Therapy*, 2 (1962), 178-705.

Bychowski, G. "The Structure of Homosexual Acting Out." *Psychoanalytic Quarterly*, 23 (1954), 48-61.

Byrd, R. *Alone*. New York: Putnam's Sons, 1938.

Carpenter, E. *The Intermediate Sex*. New York: M. Kennerly Co., 1912.

Cavan, R. S., P. M. Houser, and S. A. Stouffer. "A Note on the Statistical Treatment of Life-History Material." *Social Forces*, 30:9, 200-205.

Cartwright, D. and J. P. R. French Jr. "The Reliability of Life-History Studies." *Character and Personality*, 8 (1939), 110-119.

Chassan, J. B. "Stochastic Models of the Single Case as the Basis of Clinical Research Design." *Behavioral Science*, 6:1 (1961), 42-50.

Chein, I. *The Road to H.* New York: Basic Books, 1964.

Chessick, R. "The Pharmacogenic Orgasm in the Drug Addict." *Arch. of General Psychiatry*, 3 (April, 1960), 545-556.

Clausen, A. "Social and Psychological Factors in Narcotics Addiction." *Law and Contemporary Problems*, 22: 42.

Clinard, M. *Sociology of Deviant Behavior*. New York: Holt, Rinehart, and Winston, 1963.

Cohen, A. *Deviance and Control*. New Jersey: Prentice-Hall, 1966.

______. "The Sociology of the Deviant Act: Anomie Theory and Beyond." *American Sociological Review*, 30 (1965), 12.

Conwell, C. *The Professional Thief by A Professional Thief.* Ed. E. Sutherland. Chicago: Chicago University Press, 1937.

Cooley, C. "The Roots of Social Knowledge." *American Journal of Sociology*, 32 (July, 1926), 59-79.

Coser, L. "Some Functions of Deviant Behavior and Normative Flexibility." *American Journal of Sociology*, 68, 172-181.

Cousins, N. *Who Speaks for Man*? New York: Macmillan, 1953.

Cressey, D. "Changing Criminals: The Application of Theory of Differential Association." *American Journal of Sociology*, 61 (Sept., 1955), 116-120.

Cummings, Elaine and W. E. Henry. *Growing Old.* New York: Basic Books, 1961.

Daniels, A. and R. Daniels. "The Social Function of the Career Fool." *Psychiatry*, 27 (Aug., 1964), 219-229.

Davis, K. "The Sociology of Prostitution." *American Sociological Review*, 2 (Oct., 1937), 744-755.

Dda, C. F. "Psychological States Resulting From Para-Thyroid Deficiency." *Journal of Abnormal Social Psychology*, 34 (1939), 481-496.

Dean, D. "Alienation: Its Meaning and Measurement." *American Sociological Review*, 30 (1965), 12.

Dentler, R. "The Functions of Deviant Groups." *Social Problems*, 7 (1959), 98-107.

Devereux, G. and Bert Kaplan, ed. *Studying Personality Cross Culturally*. Elmsford, New York: Row Peterson and Co., 1961.

Dollard, J. *Criteria for the Life History.* New York: Peter Smith Co., 1949.

Durkheim, E. *The Division of Labor in Society.* New York: Glencoe Free Press, 1949.

Eidsun, Bernice T. *Scientists: Their Psychological World.* New York: Basic Books, 1962.

Eitinger. L. "Concentration Camp Survivors in the Postwar World. *American Journal of Orthopsychiatry.* 32:3 (1962), 367-375.

Erikson, E. "Identity and the Life Cycle." *Psychological Issues* 1:1 (1959).

Engel, Mary, and S. J. Blatt. "Clinical Inference in Psychological Assessment." Paper read at the American Psychological Association convention, Philadelphia. 1963.

Feifel, H., ed. *The Meaning of Death.* New York: McGraw-Hill, 1959.

Felix, R. H. "One Appraisal of the Personality Type of the Addict." *American Journal of Psychology,* 100 (1954).

Fenichel, O. *The Psychoanalytic Theory of Neurosis.* New York: Norton, 1950.

Folett, M. P. *Creative Experience.* New York: Fongmans, Green, and Co., 1924.

Frankl, V. *A Psychologist Experiences the Concentration Camp.* Vienna, 1946.

Freeman, G. L., and G. E. Manson. "The Stress Interview." *Journal of American Social Psychology,* 37 (1942), 427-447.

French, T. *The Integration of Behavior*, Vols. 1-3. Chicago: University of Chicago Press, 1952-1958.

Frenkel, E. "Studies in Biographical Psychology." *Character and Personality*, 5 (1936), 1-34.

Freud, Sigmund. "Analysis of a Phobia in a Five-Year-Old Boy" (1925A). In *Collected Papers of Sigmund Freud*, Vol. 3, 149-289. London: Hogarth Press, 1925.

______. *Beyond the Pleasure Principle*. London: Hogarth Press, 1942.

______. "The Etiology of Hysteria" (1896A). In *The Standard Edition of the Complete Psychological Works of Sigmund Freud*. London: Hogarth Press, 1962.

______. *Inhibitions, Symptoms, and Anxiety*. London: Hogarth Press, 1938.

______. *New Introductory Lectures on Psycho-Analysis*. New York: Norton, 1944.

______. *Three Essays on the Theory of Sexuality*. London: Imago, 1905.

Fried, E. *On Love and Sexuality*. New York: Grove Press, 1961.

Fromm, E. "Individual and Social Origins of Neurosis." *American Sociological Review*, 9 (1944), 380-384.

Galton, F. "Measurement of Character" *Fortnightly Review*, 36 (1844), 179-185.

Garraty, J. A. *The Nature of Biography*. New York: Knopf, 1957.

Gendlin, E. *Experiencing and the Creation of Meaning*. New York: Glencoe Free Press, 1962.

Gertzel, V., and Mildred G. Gertzel. *Cradles of Eminence.* Boston: Little, Brown, 1962.

Gerver, I., and J. Bensman. "Crime and Punishment in The Factory: A Functional Analysis." *Mass Society in Crisis.* New York: MacMillan Co., 1964.

Gesell, A. *The Mental Growth of the Pre-School Child.* New York, 1925.

Giddens, Anthony. *New Rules of Sociological Method: A Positive Critique of Interpretative Sociologies.* New York: Basic Books, 1976.

Goffman, Erving. "The Moral Career of the Mental Patient." *Psychiatry: Journal for the Study of Interpersonal Processes,* Vol. 22 (May, 1959), 123-137.

Goffman, I. *Stigma.* New Jersey: Prentice-Hall, 1963.

Gollwitzer, H., et al., eds. *Dying We Live.* New York: Pantheon, 1956.

Gottschalk, L., C. Kluchhon, and R. Angell. *The Use of Personal Documents in History, Anthropology and Sociology.* New York: Social Science Research Council, 1945.

Gruhle, H. "Selbstbiographie und Personlickkeitsforchung." *Kongress f. Experimental Psychology,* 8, 1928, 165-167.

Guthrie, E. *Psychology of Human Conflict.* New York: Hayer, 1938.

Hachiya, M. *Hiroshima Diary.* University of North Carolina, 1955.

Hall, G. S. *Adolescence.* Appleton, NY: 1904.

Hartmann, H. "Psychoanalysis as a Scientific Theory." *Psychoanalysis, Scientific Method, and Philosophy.* New York: New York University Press, 1959.

Hathaway, S. R. and J. C. McKinley. *Minnesota Multiphasic Personality Inventory.* University of Minnesota, 1942.

Healy, W. "The Contributions of Case Studies to Sociology." *American Sociological Society Publications,* 18, 147-155.

______, and Augusta Bronner. *Judge Baker Foundation Case Studies.* University of Chicago Press, 1945.

Henry, Jules. *Culture Against Man.* Vintage, 1963.

Hirsch, J. "Behavior Genetics and Individuality Understood." *Science,* 142 (1963), 1436-1442.

Hoffman, M. "Drug Addiction and Hypersexuality: Related Modes of Mastery." *Comprehensive Psychiatry,* 5:4 (August, 1964).

Hollingshead, A. B., and F. C. Redlich. "Social Stratification and Psychiatric Disorders." *Americam Sociological Review,* 18 (April, 1953), 163-169.

Holt, R. R. "An Inductive Method of Analyzing Defense of Self-Esteem." *Bull. Menninger Clin.,* 15 (1951), 6-15.

______. "Clinical Judgement as a Disciplined Inquiry." *Journal of Mental Disorders,* 133 (1961), 369-382.

______. "Individuality and Generalization in the Psychology of Personality." *Journal of Personality,* 30 (1962).

Huxley, A. *Tomorrow, and Tomorrow, and Tomorrow.* New York: Signet Books, 1956.

Jackson, D. D., ed. *The Etiology of Schizophrenia.* New York: Basic Books, 1960.

James, W. *Pragmatism.* New York: Green and Co., 1907.

______. *The Varieties of Religious Experience.* New York: Modern Library, 1902.

Johnson, A. "Sanctions for Superego Lacunae of Adolescents." Paper delivered at the Chicago Analytic Society on March 25, 1947.

Jones, E. *The Life Work of Sigmund Freud,* Vol. 2. New York: Basic Books, 1955.

Jones, S. E. In *Personality and The Behavior Disorders.* J. Hunt Ed. New York: Ronald, 1944.

Jourard, S. *The Transparent Self.* New York: D. Van Nostrand and Co., 1964.

Jung, C. G. *The Integration of Personality.* New York: Farrar and Rinehart, Inc., 1938.

Kahle, M. "Beziehungen Weiblicher Fursurgezoglinge Zur Familie." *Beihefte Z. Zsch. F. Angew Psychol,* 60 (1931), 188.

Keller, Helen. *The Story of My Life.* New York: Doubleday, 1903.

Kelley, G. A. *The Psychology of Personality Constructs.* New York: Norton, 1955.

Keniston, K. *The Uncommitted: Alienated Youth in American Society.* New York: Harcourt, Brace, and World, 1965.

Kinsey, A, and W. B. Pomeroy. *Sexual Behavior in the Human Male.* Philadelphia: Saunders, 1948.

Klapp, O. *Heroes, Villians, and Fools.* New Jersey: Prentice-Hall, 1962.

Knupfer, G. "Portrait of an Underdog." *Public Opinion Quarterly,* 11 (Spring, 1947), 103.

Korn, R. "Psychopathology as Experience and Action." Unpublished paper, School of Criminology, University of California, Berkeley.

Kraepelin, E. *Psychiatrae.* Leipzig: Barth, 1904.

Krafft-Ebing, R. *Psychopathia Sexualis.* Stuttgart: Enke, 1881.

Krueger, E. T. *Autobiographical Documents and Personality.* Chicago: Chicago University Library, 1925.

Krueger, E. and W. Reckless. *Social Psychology.* New York: Longmans, 1931.

Laing, R. D. *The Politics of the Family.* New York: Pantheon, 1971.

Lazarus, R. S. *Adjustment and Personality.* New York: McGraw-Hill, 1961.

Leary, T. *Interpersonal Diagnosis and Personality.* New York: Ronald Press, 1957.

Lederer, W. "Dragons, Delinquents, and Destiny." *Psychological Issues,* 4:3, Monograph No. 15. New York: International University Press, 1964.

Lemert, E. *Human Deviance, Social Problems and Social Control.* New Jersey: Prentice-Hall, 1967.

______. *Social Pathology.* New York: McGraw-Hill, 1951.

Levy, N. A. "An Investigation into the Nature of the Therapeutic Process: A Preliminary Report." In *Psychoanalysis and Social Process,* Vol. 4. Ed. J. H. Masserman. New York: Grune and Stratton, 1961.

Lindesmith, A. "Dope Fiend Mythology." *Journal of Criminal Law, Criminology, and Political Science,* 31:2 (July-August, 1940), 199-208.

Louttit, C. M. *Clinical Psychology.* New York: Harper and Row, 1947.

Lundber, G. "Case Work and the Statistical Method." *Social Forces,* 5 (1926).

Lustman, S. L. "Defense, Symptom, and Character." *Psychoanalytic Study of the Child,* Vol. 17. New York: International University Press, 1962.

Lyman, Stanford. L. and M. Scott. "On Accounts." Unpublished paper, Sonoma State College, California.

Machover, K. *Personality Projection.* Illinois: Chas. C. Thomas, 1949.

Marx, Karl. *Das Kapital.* New York: Chas. H. Kerr and Co., 1906.

Maslow, A. H. *Motivation and Personality.* New York: Harper and Bros., 1954.

Matza, D. *Delinquency and Drift.* New York: John Wiley and Sons, 1964.

Mead, George H. "The Psychology of Punitive Justice." American Journal of Sociology, 23 (1928), 577-602.

______. "The Social Self." *The Journal of Philosophic, Psychologic, and Scientific Methods,* 10 (1913), 375-380.

Meier, D. and W. Bell. "Anomie and Differential Access to the Achievement of Life Goals." *American Sociological Review,* 24 (April, 1959).

Mendelson, J. H., P. Kubzanshy, H. Liederman, D. Wexler, and P. Soloman. *Physiological and Psychological Aspects of Sensory Deprivation: A Case Analysis.* Harvard University Press, 1961.

Menninger, K. *A Manual for Psychiatric Case Study.* New York: Guren Stratton, 1952.

______. *The Vital Balance.* New York: Viking, 1963.

Merton, R. "Anomie, Anomia, and Social Interaction: Contexts of Deviant Behavior." In *Anomie and Deviant Behavior.* New York: Glencoe Free Press, 1964, 226.

Miller, P. R. "The Effeminate Passive Obligatory Homosexual." *A.M.A. Archives of Neurology and Psychology,* 89 (1958), 612-618.

______. "Lower Class Culture as a Generating Milieu of Gang Delinquency." *Journal of Social Issues.*

Minuchin, S. "Structured Family Therapy." *American Handbook on Psychiatry,* Vol. 3 (1972).

Murphey, G. "The Current Impact of Freud on American Psychology." *American Psychologist,* 2 (1963), 663.

Murray, H. A. et al. *Explorations in Personality: A Clinical and Experimental Study of Fifty men of College Age.* New York: Oxford University Press, 1938.

______. *Thematic Apperception Test.* Cambridge: Harvard University Press, 1943.

Nettler, G. "A Measure of Alienation." *American Sociological Review*, 22 (December, 1957).

Neugarten, Bernice L. "Personality Changes During the Adult Years." *Conference on Adult Education*. Syracuse University, October 2; 1962.

______., and Ruth J. Kraines. "Factors Related to the Mental Health of Women in the Climacteric Years." Paper delivered at the American Psychological Association convention, St. Louis, 1962.

Nunberg, H. *Principles of Psychoanalysis*. International University Press, 1955.

Parsons, Talcott. *The Social System*. New York: Glencoe Free Press, 1951.

Piaget, J. *The Origins of Intelligence in Children*. New York: International University Press, 1952.

______. *The Construction of Reality in the Child*. New York: Basic Books, 1954.

Pigors. *Case Method in Human Relations*. New York: McGraw-Hill Boók Co., 1961.

Pittenger, R., Hackett, and J. Danehy. *The First Five Minutes*. New York: Paul Martineau Publishers, 1960.

Plummer, Ken. *Documents of Life: An Introduction to the Problems and Literature of a Humanistic Method.* Boston: Allen and Unwin, 1983.

Polansky, N. A. "How Shall a Life-History Be Written?" *Character and Personality*, 9 (1941), 188-207.

Rank, O. *Modern Education*. New York: Knopf, 1932.

Reiner, B. S., and I. Kaufman. *Character Disorders in Parents of Delinquents*. New York: Family Service

Association of America, 1959.

Reiss, A. "The Social Integration of Peers and Queers." *Social Problems,* 9 (1962), 102-120.

Richard, R. W. *Modern Clinical Psychology.* New York: McGraw-Hill, 1946.

Ricouer, Paul. *Freud and Philosophy: An Essay on Interpretation.* Trans. Denis Savage. New Haven, Yale University Press, 1970.

Riley, M. *Sociological Research.* New York: Harcourt, Brace, and World, 1963.

Roe, Anne. "A Psychologist Examines 64 Eminent Scientists." *Scientific American,* 4 (1952), 87.

Rosenbloom, J. R. "Notes on Jewish Drug Addicts." *Psychological Reports,* 5 (1959), 769-772.

Rosenzweig, S. "Investigating and Appraising Personality." In *Methods of Psychology.* Ed. T. G. Andrews. New York: Wiley Press, 1948.

Rotter, J. B. "The Incomplete Sentence Test as a Method of Studying Personality." *Journal of Consulting Psychology,* 11:3 (1947), 48.

Sarbin, R. "Role Theoretical Interpretations of Psychological Change." In *Personality Change.* Ed. Worchel et al. New York: Wiley and Co., 1964.

Sarton, M. *As We Are Now.* New York: Norton, 1973.

Sartre, Jean-Paul. *Being and Nothingness.* New York: Washington Square Press, 1966.

Satir, Virginia. *Conjoint Family Therapy.* Palo Alto: Science and Behavioral Books, 1967.

Savitt, R. A. "Psychoanalytic Studies on Addiction: Ego Structure in Narcotic Addiction." *Psychoanalytic Quarterly*. (November, 1957), 43-57.

Schafer, R. *The Clinical Application of Psychological Tests*. New York: International University Press, 1965.

Schofield, M. *Sociological Aspects of Homosexuality*. Boston: Little, Brown, and Co., 1965.

Seeman, M. "On the Meaning of Alienation." *American Sociological Review*, 24 (December, 1959), 783-791.

Sennet and Cobbs, *The Hidden Injuries of Class*. New York: Vintage, 1973.

Schaffer, G. W., and L. S. Lazarus. *Fundamental Concepts in Clinical Psychology*. New York: McGraw-Hill, 1952.

Shaw, C. R. "The Case Study Technique: Value of a Delinquent Boy's Own Story." In *The Sociology of Crime and Delinquency*. Ed. M. Wolstang, L. Savitz, and N. Johnston. New York: Wiley, 1962.

Shaw, C. *The Jackroller*. Chicago: University of Chicago Press, 1939.

Sheehy, Gail. *Passages*. New York: Dutton, 1974.

Sheffield, Ada E. *The Social Case History*. New York: Sage Foundation, 1920.

Sheidman, E. S. and N. L. Farberow, eds. *Clues to Suicide*. New York: Blakiston, 1957.

Sheldon, W. and S. Stevens. *The Varieties of Temperament*. New York: Harper and Bros., 1942.

Silverberg, W. *Childhood Experiences and Personal Destiny*. New York: Springer, 1952.

Skolnick, J. *Justice Without Trial.* New York: Wiley and Sons, 1966.

Smelser and Smelser. *Personality and Social System.* New York: Wiley and Sons, 1963.

Sperle, H. *The Case Study Method Technique in Professional Training.* New York, 1933.

Srole, L. "Social Integration and Certain Corollaries: An Exploratory Study." *American Sociological Review,* 21 (1956), 709-716.

Stein, M. I. "The Use of a Sentence Completion Test for the Diagnosis of Personality." *Journal of Clinical Psychology,* 3 (1947), 46-56.

Stephenson, W. *The Study of Behavior.* Chicago: University of Chicago Press, 1953.

Stern, W. *Anfange der Reifezeit.* Leipzig, 1925.

______. *Intelligenz der Kinder und Jugendlichen.* Leipzig, 1929.

Stinchcombe, Arthur L. *Theoretical Methods in Social History.* New York: Academic Press, 1978.

Straus, E. W. "The Sigh: An Introduction to a Theory of Expressions." *Tijdschrift Voor Philosophie,* 14 (1952), 1-22.

Strupp, H. H., and L. Luborsky, eds. *Research on Psycho-Therapy.* Washington, D. C.: American Psychological Association, 1962.

Sullivan, H. S. *Interpersonal Theory of Psychiatry.* New York: Norton, 1953.

______. "The Meaning of Anxiety in Psychiatry and in Life." *Psychiatry* 11:1 (1948).

Sussman, L. "F. D. R. and The White House Mail." *Public Opinion Quarterly,* 20 (1956), 5-16.

Sutherland, E. H. *The Professional Thief.* Chicago: University of Chicago Press, 1937.

Symonds, P. M. "The Sentence Completion Test as a Projective Technique." *Journal of Abnormal and Social Psychology,* 42 (1947), 320-329.

Szurek, S. "Genesis of Psychopathic Personality Trends." *Psychiatry,* 5 (1942), 1.

Taft, J. "Thirty-One Contacts With a Seven Year Old Boy." In *Dynamics of Therapy.* New York: MacMillan, 1933.

Taylor, Charles. "Interpretation and the Sciences of Man." *Review of Metaphysics,* 25:1 (September, 1971).

Thomas, W. I. and F. Znaniecki. "Life Record of an Immigrant." *The Polish Peasant in Europe and America,* Vol. 2. New York: Knopf, 1927.

Thompson, C. "Changing Concepts of Homosexuality in Psychoanalysis." *Psychiatry,* 10 (1947), 2-13.

Thrasher, F. *The Gang.* Chicago: University of Chicago Press, 1927.

Turner, Ralph. "Role-Taking, Role Standpoint, and Reference-group Behavior." *American Journal of Sociology,* 61 (January, 1956), 316- 328.

Viorst, J. *Necessary Losses.* New York: Simon and Schuster, 1986.

Vogel, E. and N. Bell., eds. "The Emotionally Disturbed Child as the Family Scapegoat." In *The Family.* New York: Glencoe Free Press, 1962.

Watson, R. *The Clinical Method in Psychology*. New York: Harper and Row, 1951.

Weil, A. and W. Rosen. *Chocolate to Morphine*. Houghton-Mifflin Co., 1983.

Wells, H. G. *Experiment in Autobiography*. New York: MacMillan, 1934.

Wheelis, A. B. *The Quest for Identity*. New York: Norton, 1958.

Whyte, W. F. *Street Corner Society: The Social Structure of an Italian Slum*. Chicago: University of Chicago Press, 1943.

Wiesel, E. *The Jews of Silence*. New York: Signet, 1967.

Wilkins, L. *Social Deviance*. New Jersey: Prentice-Hall, 1965.

______. "Information and Decisions Regarding Offenders." Unpublished paper, School of Criminology, University of California, Berkeley.

Wittels, F. *Sigmund Freud*. London: Allen and Unwin, 1924.

Witwer, Helen L. "Increasing the Research Value of Case Records." *Sociology and Social Research,* 15 (November, 1939), 116-125.

Wood, Vivian. and Bernice L. Neugarten. "Social Role Change and Mental Health in the Climacteric Years." Paper read at the American Sociological Association meetings, Washington, 1962.

Wylie, P. *Generation of Vipers*. New York: Farrar and Rinehart, 1942.

Zigler, E. and L. Phillips. "Psychiatric Diagnosis and Symptomatology." *Journal of Abnormal Psychology and Sociology*, 62:1 (July, 1961).

## Author Index

Martin Grotjahn

## MY FAVORITE PATIENT

The Memoirs of a Psychoanalyst

Psychopathologie und Humanwissenschaften. Vol. 2

ISBN 3-8204-5648-1 302 pages paperback US $ 47.20 / sFr. 66.00

Recommended prices – alterations reserved

The author shows on his personal and his professional life story the development of a person and of an analyst. His idea all through life was always to look at himself as if he was his own favorite patient – and at his patients as if they were himself, or at least parts of himself. This development is traced through childhood, medical school, marriage, emigration, war experience, and finally through the life of an analyst in Beverly Hills, Southern California, USA. The story is told with humor, illustrated by approximately 50 drawings by the author himself. He shows his increasing insight, his understanding for himself and others; his deepening maturation as a person and simultaneously as a therapist.

Contents: Born in Berlin in 1904, took his medical and psychoanalytic training there in Berlin – Emigrated in September 1936 and analyzed within himself what it means to get married, and become a father, to mature as a person, as a physician, and as a therapist.

PETER LANG PUBLISHING, INC.
62 West 45th Street
USA – New York, NY 10036

Marlene Christine Mills

## Adolescent Self-Disclosure

Its Facilitation Through Themes, Therapeutic Techniques and Interview Conditions

American University Studies: Series VIII (Psychology). Vol. 3
ISBN 0-8204-0115-3 188 pp. hardback US $ 23.50/sFr. 54.00

Recommended prices - alterations reserved

How might an adolescent be facilitated to self-disclose in a counselling interview? This research undertook the task of studying this rather neglected area in the literature on adolescents, psychotherapy, and self-disclosure. Adolescents, and in particular those with learning difficulties and/or behavior problems, are in need of methods to facilitate self-expression. The major purpose of this research was to verify the efficacy of three factors facilitating self-divulgence: psychotherapeutic techniques, individual and group conditions, and themes. The findings responded to how adolescents may be facilitated to self-disclose.

Contents: Adolescent self-disclosure - Inhibitive and facilitative aspects of individual and group counselling conditions - Theme-centered interviews - Positive and negative characteristics of therapeutic techniques - Measurement of self-disclosure.

PETER LANG PUBLISHING, INC.
62 West 45th Street
USA - New York, NY 10036